INTERMITTENT FASTING
FASTING
for *Women Over* 50

The Ultimate Guide to Reset Your Metabolism, Accelerate Weight Loss, Detox Your Body and Start Enjoying a Healthier and Happier Life!

CORI KIMBERLEIGH

Table of Contents

Introduction

Congratulations on purchasing *Intermittent Fasting For Women Over 50,* and thank you for doing so. A woman's body makes drastic changes after approaching 50 years of age, including changes in the metabolism, body, and the onset of menopause. Even though mother nature has all of the control, there are some things you can do to slow the process.

> *"Winning and losing isn't everything. Sometimes, the journey is just as important as the outcome."*

Alex Morgan

Alex Morgan knows what she is talking about. You learn a lot about yourself as you begin a new dieting plan - the pros and cons of your dieting behavior.

Fasting isn't a trend and has been a part of some religious beliefs, including Islam, Hinduism, Buddhist fasting, Orthodox Christian fasting, and others. Decades before this generation, the process may have been because of the unavailability of food resources. Just remember, it is not a starvation diet since starvation is considered an involuntary absence of food. Consider breakfast as the most crucial time of your day. After all, *'break-fast'* is a part of every day.

Suppose you vary your fasting period too much. In that case, it can lead to an erratic change in your hormones, which among other things, makes it much more difficult for your body to shed any excess weight. If you find yourself without the time required to eat a proper meal to break the fast, ensure you at least eat something to keep your body on the appropriate keto cycle.

While the core ideas behind the various forms of intermittent fasting are generally the same, there are many ways to go about it. Your best bet is to try a few and see which one your body naturally responds to the easiest. Just remember not to cut the calories too much in the beginning.

Intermittent fasting can provide many benefits, which you will discover in-depth in future chapters. First, let's explore how a woman's body reacts to aging.

> *"Let food be thy medicine,*
> *and medicine be thy food."*
>
> Hippocrates

So, if you found this book useful in any way, a review on Amazon is always appreciated!

Chapter 1

Introduction to IF
With Scientific Proof

Intermittent fasting is backed up by science. Your metabolic rate is increased with short-term fasting because of the hormonal changes ranging from 3.6% to 14%. Studies have established weight loss after three to twenty-four weeks on the intermittent fasting program to maintain losses of 3.0 to 8.0%. In comparison to other studies on weight loss, these are high percentages you cannot ignore.

In the same studies, many individuals lost 4.0 to 7.0% of his/her waist circumference. This progress indicates how the harmful buildup of belly fat can cause disease and other issues around your organs. You have to consider these results from eating fewer calories and not binging during the days off.

You have to maintain a sensible eating program. Intermittent fasting is a way of eating to ensure that you get the most out of every meal you eat. The core tenants of intermittent fasting mean that you don't need to change what you are eating; instead, you have to change *when* eating it.

Intermittent fasting is a viable alternative to traditional diets or merely cutting your daily caloric intake.

Intermittent fasting is also an excellent option for those who traditionally have trouble sticking to diet plans. It only requires you to change one small habit instead of several larger ones. Intermittent fasting is beneficial for most people because it is simple enough for them to attempt - yet sufficient enough to warrant doing it. The key to understanding why intermittent fasting is so successful - lies in your body's differences during a fasted state versus a fed state. These essential changes will come across with changing habits and sticking with the techniques used.

The body is considered to be in the fed state when it is absorbing and digesting food. The fed state tends to start roughly five minutes after you begin eating and lasts for three to five hours, depending on how long it takes your body to digest the meal. A "fed state" leads to higher insulin levels, making it much more difficult for the body to burn fat. The period directly after the "fed state" is referred to as the postabsorptive state, which is the 'time' where the body is not actively processing food. Its insulin levels begin to fall. This state lasts for between eight and twelve hours and directly precedes the fasted state.

The fasted state occurs between nine and twelve hours after the postabsorptive state. It is the point where the body's insulin levels are at their lowest, making it the time where the most fat - might be burned during physical activity. Unfortunately, many rarely go twelve hours without eating, which means that no matter how hard they exercise, they do not burn fat as efficiently as possible. However, this also means that you can burn fat and build muscle by altering your feeding habits.

While the science behind intermittent fasting is certainly promising, there are a few things you will need to keep in mind when starting any new dietary plan. No diet, regardless of how miraculous it appears, can help you - if you don't obey a few general rules, you will discover throughout this guideline. *The hard days are what make you stronger*", according to Aly Raisman.

Reach Ketosis

Using a ketogenic diet plan, you will achieve what's called - ketosis. The dieting method will allow you to lower your calorie intake below the caloric volume your body can consume each day. Thus, it is vital to summon the energy stored in the fat cells to send fuel or power to your muscles - accomplished through the dieting technique used by the keto diet, limiting the volume of carbs you consume.

A substantial percentage of your fuel for the day will come from fat transformed to ketones. After you have the carbohydrates, protein, and fat ratio monitored, you're well on the way to a successful diet strategy. You won't be over-eating with large portions of protein. You also won't eliminate fat or carbs, making it a safe diet plan for fat loss.

Suppose you take the approach of eating less without considering your diet. In that case, you'll be losing the essential vitamins and minerals needed daily - possibly resulting in fatigue, muscle spasms, mental fogginess, headaches, hunger, irritability, emotional depression, or insomnia. You can also lose valuable muscle mass, not just the pounds you intended to drop.

Using the enclosed low-carb dieting plan, you can lower your intake of carbohydrates, reduce your calorie counts, and nurture your body with a sufficient supply of water, eggs, meat, fish, veggies, high-quality oils, and nuts which can help drop the pounds without any bothersome side effects.

The huge plus, of course, is that you lose weight, but you will also lower your triglycerides, blood pressure, and blood sugar. There's no set rule for carb intake. These are the basic guidelines to consider as you blaze the path to weight loss:

- *100-150 Grams Each Day*: Stay within these limits if you are active and lean, trying to maintain weight.

- *20-50 Grams Each Day*: If you have diabetes, are obese, or are metabolically deranged, this is the plan for you. Your body will achieve a ketosis state which supplies the ketone bodies.

As you now see, it is important to experiment and categorize where you fall on the scales before you make any changes. As with any new diet changes, you should seek your doctor's advice.

Each individual will lose weight differently, and other people may not have the same goals as you. For now, as a beginner, you will be using the first method. These are four unique plans, so you better understand the different levels:

Ketogenic Technique #1: The standard ketogenic diet (SKD) consists of moderate protein, high-fat, and is low in carbs.

Ketogenic Technique #2: Workout times will call for the targeted keto diet, also called TKD. The process consists of adding additional carbohydrates to the diet plan when you are more active.

Ketogenic Technique #3: The cyclical ketogenic diet (CKD) entails a restricted five-day keto diet plan followed by two high-carbohydrate days.

Ketogenic Technique #4: The high-protein keto diet is comparable to the standard keto plan (SKD) in all aspects, except you will consume more protein.

*"Start where you are. Use what you have.
Do what you can. After all, the journey is
worth the challenges."*

Arthur Ashe

How You Are Affected By Menopause

Your Metabolism Slows Down: The main element to remember is you need to take in fewer calories.

Your Brain May Weaken: Your brain is much like a muscle. You must use it, or it will become weak and shrink. Do new things in your life and step out of your comfort zone. It pushes your brain into an active mode when you switch things up. It could be as simple as going down a different path on the way home or changing the way you eat! Break the routine and try intermittent fasting to help slow the aging process.

Your Short-Term Memory Changes: Have you ever been around an individual who is over 50? If you are close with that person, you may notice some of the short-term memories will begin to fade, which can impact your daily routines. It's often displayed in the form of slowed reaction times and poor judgment.

Your Eyesight May Deteriorate or Weaken: As you age, the darkness may be your worst enemy, which increases the issues involved with depth and distance perception. It's probably not to drive except during daylight hours. It's essential to take care of your eyesight and visit your optician regularly.

Your Bone Loss Accelerates: The menopause time brings forth acceleration for three to five years, leading to bone fractures, many times brought on by a fall. Workout using your major muscle groups for some improvement of bone protection. Try working out a couple of times each week.

Your Muscle Loss Accelerates: Your peak of muscle mass generally occurs at the age of 25. After 50, the loss of hormones, such as the growth hormone, is reduced. Make adequate sleeping a goal since that's when your hormones are released. Opt for short intervals and weight training, working hard at short intervals, "hit it and quit it!"

You Are More Susceptible to Injuries: You don't think about injuries at 50 because your mindset still thinks it's as agile now as it was at 21. Unfortunately, you're more likely to suffer from medical issues like carpal tunnel syndrome, tendinitis, and plantar fasciitis. It's recommended to take frequent breaks if you're at a work desk all day. Exercise is the key, so stretch your forearms or develop another inventive way to keep your muscles active to avoid so many repetitive movements.

You Lose Flexibility: Don't try to do the splits as you did in your younger years. Your tendons and muscles lose their elasticity. Your spinal discs will also degenerate with age, raising your chances of injuries. You may need to use alternative healthcare as part of your health regimen. Consider chiropractic care, massage therapy, and stretching exercises.

Lactose Intolerance Becomes An Issue: Milk is considered the #1 calcium supplier for strong and healthy bones. Aging can bring forth problems with women digesting milk properly as she ages. Intermittent fasting can add back some of the calcium by providing your diet with leafy greens, Greek yogurt, hard cheese, kefir, and tofu.

Hormonal Changes May Prompt Digestive Issues: As hormones change, expect the menopause changes (on average) by 51. It's possible you will suffer from gas, bloating, and constipation.

Your Fat Will Redistribute: During child-bearing years, the woman's body has fat allocated to her thighs and hips to support carrying a child. That changes during menopause as the body produces less estrogen; the fat collects in the tummy area, called 'menopause belly.'

Your Body Stores More Fat: Aging causes your body to store fat readily and reluctantly burns fat, especially if you are dehydrated or stressed. Estrogen dropping adds to the adverse effects of stress. It also deviates the fat from reproductive areas. Thus, you gain weight around the belly - losing your hourglass figure. The intermittent fasting methods will assist you by providing snacks and treats to enjoy using the ketogenic dieting methods. Provide extra fiber and protein to reduce your cravings and keep you satiated longer.

You Are More Prone To Calcium Deficiency: Your bones are weakened when calcium is depleted. The lack of calcium can lead to bone pain and tenderness or osteoporosis. You should ingest 1200 mg. of calcium daily. Once again, intermittent fasting using cheese and yogurt are excellent remedies. Other calcium-rich foods include kidney beans, kale, broccoli, oranges, sesame seeds, edamame, and almonds.

Your Body Synthesizes Protein Less Effectively: After 50, it's essential to consume adequate protein in your diet, or muscle loss may result. Strength training can improve the process, so it's vital to enjoy a high-protein meal about one or two hours after you have your workout.

You Might Develop Dry Mouth: With aging, the possibilities of diabetes, high blood pressure, arthritis, and Parkinson's, many individuals suffer from dry mouth brought on by many of the popular medications used to treat the ailment. Dry mouth can also lead to fungal infections of the throat, tongue, and other areas, including tooth decay and gum disease. Drink lots of water to stay hydrated, ensuring you floss regularly to remove plaque and food possibly stuck in your teeth.

You'll Have More Dental Issues: By the age of 50, enamel erodes, creating an increase in dental issues that may require increased care to eliminate tooth pain and unwanted cavities. It's vital to have regular dental exams and stop some of the woes after 50!

You May Develop Foot Conditions: Some individuals will have deformities, including bunions and hammertoes, as a part of the aging process. In some cases, they are hereditary. Choose a good-fitting shoe that's not too tight to dissuade the worsening of the problem.

Your Feet Will Change Shape: It sounds crazy, but you may notice your feet become wider or longer during the aging process. According to Dr. Petkov, a podiatrist in New Jersey, *"They can grow half a size in a decade."* Your feet can also become flat since the ligaments and tendons lose their resilience. You will find that weight is a huge factor. It's essential to have someone measure your feet every few years to ensure that you are buying the right shoe size.

Your Hair & Nails Become Stressed: It's vital to increase your calcium intake because, like your skin, your hair and nails also change. You may notice your nails are brittle, and your hair has a bunch of split ends.

Your Skin Changes: You will experience a lack of estrogen, which affects your skin, making it have the appearance of cellulite more prevalent and crepe-like. You can use a remedy on the intermittent fasting plan. Have a bit of bone broth or a dash of collagen powder to a cup of coffee or smoothie.

Your Libido Declines As You Go Through Menopause: Get plenty of sleep and opt for strength training a couple of times each week. You should also perform short interval training sessions once or twice weekly. Reducing the amount of sugar and alcohol (if you drink) you consume can boost your libido.

Now, let's see how intermittent fasting can help relieve some of the stress from the toll your body takes after you hit the 50-year marker!

Medical Disclaimer: If you have a particular disease, please consult your doctor before starting this diet.

"It's never too late to change old habits."

Florence Joyner

Chapter 2

Importance of Intermittent Fasting

"It's okay to struggle, but it's not okay to give up on yourself or your dreams."

Gabe Grunewald

Intermittent fasting is beneficial in many ways. All you need is the right mindset when you begin the fasting process.

Diseases Prevention

Increase Your Brain Power: IF may have remarkable advantages for your brain by increasing new neurons' growth and protecting your brain from damage.

Reduce Risk of Alzheimer's Disease: Studies in animals suggest that IF may protect against neurodegenerative diseases such as Alzheimer's disease.

Reduce Inflammation Markers In Your body: Studies show intermittent fasting can reduce oxidative damage and inflammation. That makes IF beneficial for those who are aging and have a development of numerous diseases.

Reduce Insulin Resistance & Lower Your Risk of Type 2 Diabetes: Studies have shown IF can improve an array of risk factors for heart disease, including blood pressure, inflammatory markers, triglycerides, and cholesterol levels.

Lindsey Vonn stated, *"Life changes very quickly, in a very positive way, if you let it."*

The Right Mindset

"There may be tough times, but the difficulties which you face will make you more determined", said Marta. No method of dieting will work unless you have your mind in tune with your body. Follow a few of these suggestions to start your journey.

- *Set Goals*: Start with one of the easier plans and decide how many pounds you need to lose. Decide what type of meal plan you will be using. Make a list of your goals, but make them attainable. Look at the short term while keeping the future in sight.

- *Choose How You Want to Fast*: Try one of the more uncomplicated plans to start your IF routine. If it has not proven somewhat effective, try another strategy.

- *Stick to the Routine as Much as Possible*: Timing is an essential factor when using IF. Your body has to set the pace to drop the pounds, which will make you feel much healthier.

- *Stay Hydrated*: Everyone needs to consume plenty of healthy fluids between meals.

- *Exercise Portion Control*: Try using a smaller plate to trick your mind (it works because it's my method).

- *Make Sure You Maintain A Calorie Deficit*: While this is true for any diet, it is especially true for intermittent fasting. It can be incredibly easy to overeat once you do eat in such a way that it negates any benefits you might have felt. Remember, you need to burn 3,500 calories per week to lose one pound regularly each week; it's up to you to delegate those calories.

• *Remember To Remain Consistent:* Regardless of the type of weight loss technique you choose to pursue, it is crucial to choose one and stick with it. Remember, fasting regularly and consistently is the surest way to see any of its benefits. Your body will adjust to a new routine and increase the number of positive enzymes and neural pathways to maximize weight loss using this method. Consider consistency, the 'ace-in-the-hole of proactive weight loss success.

Common Mistakes Avoided

• *Don't Use Fasting As An Excuse:* Intermittent fasting works on the principle that eating fewer calories than you burn is a surefire way to lose weight. This theory falls apart if you use the fact that you are fasting as an excuse to eat nothing but junk food when you are on the eating cycle. Self-control and self-discipline are both equally important when it comes to eating correctly. Intermittent fasting has a wide variety of health benefits. Why not accentuate them even more with a healthy diet to go along with it?

• *Maintain Self-Control:* Intermittent fasting only works if your body goes entirely without food for at least twelve hours. Any caloric intake resets the cycle. As such, it is imperative to ensure that you maintain control of your bodily urges if you hope to see real results from this type of approach. Remember, fasting for at least twelve hours will allow you to eat normally or slightly more than an average meal. The process doesn't give you a license to eat everything in sight. Keeping your appetite in check is a strict requirement for success.

"Life is about challenges
and how we face up to them."

Martina Navratilova

Test to Remain in Ketosis

According to Mia Hamm, *"I've worked too hard and too long to let anything stand in the way of my goals"* and could not have been stated better as you go through the dieting process.

It is important to test your ketone levels to remain in ketosis. As the ketones are produced in the liver, the body is shifting its metabolism away from glucose and forward to fat utilization. *Nutritional ketosis is defined by serum ketones ranging from 0.5 to 3.0 mm.*

Use A Blood Ketone Meter: The ketone bodies - beta-hydroxybutyrate or BHB - are the most accurately measured using a blood ketone meter. The meter is pricey, but it's the most accurate tool.

Use Urine Ketone Strips: Uriscan and Ketostix are not as accurate as other methods. They can only measure acetoacetate levels. They are useful in the first phase of the diet when you just seek the carbohydrate levels to enter into ketosis. On the top side, they are simple to use and start at about $7 monthly for the strips.

Use the Ketonix Acetone Breathalyzer: Your acetone is tested using this cheaper alternative. However, breath ketones don't always correlate with blood ketones since they could be affected by alcohol consumption or water intake before testing.

Chapter 3

Different Types of IF

*"I am a better person
when I have less on my plate."*

Elizabeth Gilbert

Before you get started, think of how you want to proceed with your meal plan. If you're on an eight-hour feeding window, think about this as a schedule:

- *Hour One*: Break your fast using a typical meal.
- *Hour Two:* Enjoy a small snack such as fruit.
- *Hour Three*: Eat your second to last regular meal.
- *Hour Five*: Indulge in another small snack. Consider using one of your new recipes.
- *Hour Seven*: Sit down and enjoy your last typical meal of the day.

Arrange your meal plan using a light breakfast such as a smoothie or egg serving followed by lunch and dinner. You will also be offered a dessert or snack to be consumed according to the calories or net carbs you have designed in your dieting plan.

If you are new to intermittent fasting, you may want to begin by skipping meals or use one of the chosen methods of your liking that best suits your schedule and lifestyle. Now, let's see which option you would like to use.

Skipping Meals

Skip a meal daily to start your IF routine. All you need to do is eliminate one of your large meals. Eliminate breakfast for starters unless you must have a full meal in the morning. Getting into a fasting routine is vital to see the maximum results of your effort.

What's more, once you have tried skipping a meal now and then, you can see for yourself just how easy it is to lead to more positive changes down the line. With so many intermittent fasting options available, the odds are good that one fits your schedule, so give it a try. What have you got to lose (besides a few pounds)?

Crescendo Technique

This crescendo process is excellent for women and is ranked as suitable for women since you can begin fasting without irritating your hormones or shocking any part of your body. It utilizes a fasting window of 12-16 hours. You can enjoy your meals for 8-12 hours. Space the fasting schedule out for a few days, such as Monday, Wednesday, and Friday. If you have failed other diets, this might be your answer. After two weeks, add one more day of active fasting to your schedule.

5:2 Or Fast Diet Technique

For women, just restrict calories for two days each week by having two meals (250 calories each). Men can have 600 calories or 300 calories for two meals. The rule of thumb is based on men needing 2,400 calories and women 2,000 calories. Eat as you usually do for the remainder of the week using the recipes provided in your new book. There are not that many statistics on this diet for women, but it is considered safe. Consider consuming about 1/4 of your regular calorie intake.

Soups are an excellent choice for your fasting days. These are several other examples:

- Tea
- Black coffee
- Plenty of water
- Generous portions of veggies
- Natural yogurt and berries
- Baked or boiled eggs
- Lean meat or grilled fish
- Cauliflower rice

16/8 or Leangains Technique

The name of the plan says it all, but there is an exception for women. You fast for 16 hours and eat within the 8-hour window. The scale for men is 16 hours, but it is 14 hours for women. You should only consume food with zero calories during this period, including black coffee (a splash of cream is okay), water, diet soda, and sugar-free gum. The easiest way to attempt this schedule is to stop eating after dinner in the evening and wait 14 or 16 hours from there, which means skipping breakfast and eating again in the early afternoon.

12/12 Fasting Technique

If you are a beginner, the 12-hour fast may be an excellent approach for you since the fasting window is relatively small. You are fasting as you sleep, so go ahead and sleep away many of the hunger effects of not eating.

14/10 Fasting Technique

This schedule is similar to the 16/8 method. The intermittent fasting 14/10 is very similar to that type. With this plan, you are allowed to eat whatever you want during a 10-hour window. If you get up early, you can start eating at 7 AM, and then your last meal this day will have to be at 5 PM, followed by a fasting period which will end by 7 AM the next day.

You can also have your first meal at 8 AM or 9 AM, and then your dinner will have to be no later than 6 PM and 7 PM, respectively. You can eat your usual meals during the 10-hour window, but you can't consume any calories during a 14-hour fast. However, you are allowed to drink unsweetened tea or coffee and, of course, water.

Alternate Day Diet Technique

This form of intermittent fasting means you never have to go long without food if you so choose. Every other day you should eat regularly. On the off-days, you merely consume one-fifth of the calories you usually intake on the average days.

The average daily caloric consumption is between 2,000 and 2,500 calories, which means that the regular off-day varies between 400 and 500 calories. If you enjoy exercising every day, you may need to attempt another fasting technique since you will have to severely limit your workouts on off-days.

When you first start this form of intermittent fasting, the easiest way to make it through the low-calorie days is by trying a variety of protein shakes. It is important to work back to natural foods these days because they will always be healthier than the shakes.

This form of intermittent fasting is all about losing weight. Those who try it tend to average between two and three pounds lost per week. If you attempt the Alternate Day Diet, it is critical to eat regularly on your full-calorie days. Binging will negate any progress you have made and can also cause severe damage to your body if it's continued over time.

Let's Recap

Again, when you fast, the specifics are not nearly as important as ensuring that you fast for the same time, as regularly as possible. If you vary your fasting period, it can lead to an erratic change in your hormones. This change can make it much more difficult for your body to shed excess pounds.

"Food can be both enjoyable and nourishing."

Alyssa Ardolino

If you find yourself without the time required to eat a proper meal to break your fast, you should at least eat something to keep your body on the correct cycle.

If you are exercising and intermittent fasting, it is essential to ensure that you are eating more carbohydrates than fats while you are working out. On days you are not exercising, the opposite is true. It's vital to keep your protein intake at a steady level and stay away from processed foods.

The benefits of this type of fasting are that it is incredibly flexible. It will work for a wide variety of schedules. Most people find it helpful to either eat two large meals during the eight or ten-hour feeding period or split that time into three smaller meals.

On days you are exercising and fasting, it is crucial to break your fast with a mix of protein, veggies, and fruit. Suppose you generally go to the gym after you have broken your fast. In that case, it is essential to include enough carbohydrates to give your muscles the energy they need to get the most out of your workout.

If you are planning to exercise, it is generally best to start the early afternoon off right with a medium-calorie meal. Then, exercise within three hours before eating a larger meal soon afterward. In this larger meal, it is crucial to add a larger portion of complex carbohydrates. You can even have a little dessert as long as it is in moderation. Choose one of your new recipes. Remember, fasting is different from dieting.

On days you do not plan on exercising, it is essential to adjust your caloric intake appropriately. Start by limiting your carbohydrate intake. Focus on eating lots of protein, dark green, leafy vegetables, and fruit in moderation.

Unlike on days you are exercising, the first meal you eat on rest days should be your largest - concerning your caloric intake, with this one meal counting for about 40 percent of your daily total.

Remember, during this meal, you should be taking in more protein than anything else. For your final meal during rest days, it's essential to include a protein source that will take lots of time to digest, which means it will keep you full for more of your fast the following morning. It also provides the body with enough stored amino acids to prevent it from breaking down muscle as you fast.

It is all up to you!

*"Goals should never be easy;
they should force you to work,
even if they are uncomfortable
at the time."*

Michael Phelps

Chapter 4

Foods to Include for IF

First, let's see what we should be eating to blaze your path to good health.

Dairy Options

The following list is the best for the time you are on the intermittent fasting plan. Each is low-carb and keto-friendly - listed in carbs:

- Almond milk is the #1 choice (1.4 grams per one cup).
- Coconut milk is a bit high (13 grams for one cup).
- Macadamia nut milk (one gram per cup).
- Flax milk (one gram for each cup).
- Soy milk (three net carbs per gram).
- Cashew milk (two grams of net carbs for each cup).
- Pea milk (two grams of net carbs for each cup).
- Half-and-Half is used often with a high rating of (0.6 grams of carbs per one tablespoon). If you do not have any heavy cream, substitute with this simple recipe for one cup:
    Mix whole milk (.66 or 2/3 cup)
    With melted butter (.33 or 1/3 cup)

You may be asking why you cannot have regular milk while intermittent fasting. As you age, you may be one of the many who avoid milk that contains moderate or excessive amounts of carbs. Here are several types of milk that you should avoid while

on keto with the net carbs listed for one cup:
- Cow's milk (12 grams): Cow's milk contains lactose - milk sugar - including evaporated milk, ultra-filtered milk, and raw cow's milk.
- Oat milk (17 grams): Oat milk is made from oats, which are naturally high in carbs - making oat milk inappropriate for keto.
- Goat's milk (11 grams): This is another 'bad' choice with its natural sugars, making it too high in carbs to be keto-friendly.
- Rice milk (21 grams) is naturally high in carbs.

"To ensure good health:
eat lightly, breathe deeply,
live moderately, cultivate cheerfulness,
and maintain an interest in life."

William Londen

Butter or Ghee?

You will see recipes with each of these items listed. Do you know the difference between each? You can promote fat loss and retain lean muscle mass using butter. Butter consists of water, milk solids, and butterfat.

Ghee, an Indian staple, is sometimes called clarified butter includes pure butterfat. Therefore, if you have lactose sensitivities, ghee is probably your best choice. The ghee also contains medium-chain fatty acids, which assist your immune system and digestion.

Cheese Options

Your recipes have the grams calculated, but you need to remain focused if you want to enjoy them. These are shown in net carbs:

- Soft and hard cheeses (ex. sharp cheddar or mozzarella)
- Brie Cheese - 0.1 grams - per 1 oz.
- Cheddar/Colby Cheese - 0.4 grams per 1 oz.
- Cottage cheese - creamed - 2.8 grams per .5 cup
- Cottage cheese - 2% fat - 4.1 grams per .5 cup
- Cream cheese - 0.8 grams per 2 tbsp.
- Sour cream: 1 gram per 1 tbsp.
- Parmesan cheese - 0.9 grams per 1 oz.
- Feta Cheese - 1.2 grams per 1 oz.

Cheese Recipes

Save a ton of calories and know you are consuming a low-calorie cheese product.

Almond "Feta"

Essential Ingredients:
- Olive oil (2.5 tbsp.)
- Water (.5 cup)
- Salt (1 tsp.)
- Garlic (2 minced cloves)
- Lemon juice (.25 cup)
- Cheesecloth (3 pieces)

Preparation Steps:
1. Pour the olive water, oil, salt, garlic, and lemon juice into the blender. Mix until creamy.
2. Cover a small mixing bowl using the cheesecloth before adding it to the blended mixture. Tie the cheesecloth into a ball. Set the cheese ball into a strainer and place it over the bowl. Let the cheese sit for 12 hours up to overnight.
3. Set the oven to 180° Fahrenheit/82° Celsius before adding the cheese ball onto a baking dish that has been greased.
4. Bake for about 42 minutes. Cool and use as desired.

Essential Ingredients:
- Raw cashews (.5 cup + 2 tbsp.)
- Garlic powder (1 pinch)
- Yeast (.33 cup)
- Powdered onion (1 tsp.)
- Sea salt (2 tsp.)
- Unsweetened soy milk (1.75 cups)
- Agar powder (8 tsp.)
- Lemon juice (1 tbsp.)
- Yellow/white miso (2 tbsp.)
- Canola oil (.25 cup)
- *Optional:* Truffle oil & chives
- *Also Needed:* Food processor & 3 or 4 small ramekins

Preparation Steps:
1. Brush the ramekins with oil.
2. Toss the cashews into the processor and pulse. Measure and mix in the salt, garlic powder, powdered onion, and yeast to the processor. Pulse until combined.
3. Add the oil, agar, and milk into a saucepan.
4. Once boiling, reduce the temperature setting to low-med. Simmer, covered for ten minutes. Stir thoroughly to ensure the agar is well dissolved.
5. Add the mixture to the food processor, working it steadily for two minutes until it's combined. Blend in the lemon juice, miso, and any additional flavoring fixings.
6. For sliced or grated cheese, cover the cheese and refrigerate for 4 hours until firm before removing the cheese from the ramekin using a sharp knife.
7. If it's melted cheese you're after, wait until it's hardened. Melt by placing in a saucepan to warm using medium heat. Mix in additional soy milk to achieve your desired consistency.
8. If covered and refrigerated, the cheese will keep for four days.

Serving Yields: 16 - 1 tbsp. each
Total Macro Nutrients for Each Portion:
- Net Carbs: 2.3 g
- Protein Count: 1.8 g
- Fat Content: 3 g

Essential Ingredients:
- Raw cashews (.75 cup)
- Sea salt (.75 tsp.)
- Nutritional yeast (3 tbsp.)
- Garlic powder (.25 tsp.)

Preparation Steps:
1. Add each of the fixings into a food processor.
2. Pulse until it's an ultra-fine meal.
3. Store in the fridge for two or three weeks.

<u>*Pepper Jack - Almond Milk*</u>

Essential Ingredients:
- Onion powder (.33 tsp.)
- Almond milk (12 oz./340 g - divided)
- Red pepper flakes (.33 tsp.)
- Chickpea flour (1 tbsp.)
- Agar powder (3 tsp.)
- Salt (.33 tsp.)
- Tapioca (2 tbsp.)
- Apple cider vinegar (1 tsp.)
- Garlic powder (.33 tsp.)
- Olive oil (2 tbsp.)
- Lemon juice (1 tsp.)
- Yeast (2 tbsp.)

Preparation Steps:
1. Grease the container to be used as a mold.
2. Combine the starches in a large bowl and whisk well before adding in the flour, almond milk, spices, salt, lemon juice, and oil.
3. Mix the agar and 1 cup of milk into a saucepan using medium heat. Simmer for 4 minutes past the point it begins to boil - set the temperature to low before adding the starch and almond milk.
4. Add the red pepper flakes and taste test for seasoning. It is best to overcompensate the spices. (As it solidifies, some of the flavors will be lost.)
5. Raise the heat to the medium temperature setting. Simmer and stir often for 5 minutes.
6. Stir in the red pepper flakes. Remove the pan off the burner and place it into a greased container.
7. Chill for at least one hour before grating into your recipe.

Essential Ingredients:
- Powdered agar (1.66 tbsp.)
- Water (1.66 cups)
- Onion flakes (1 tbsp.)
- Yeast (.33 cup)
- Ground dill (.33 tbsp.)
- Soaked cashews (.66 cup)
- Salt (1 pinch)
- Tahini (2 tbsp.)
- Powdered garlic (.33 tbsp.)
- Lemon (1 juiced)
- Dijon mustard (2 tsp.)

Preparation Steps:
1. Oil and set aside a storage container, ramekin, or mold of your choice.
2. Combine the cashews, lemon juice, nutritional yeast, mustard, tahini, garlic, salt, onion flakes, dill, and garlic powder. Blend until it's smooth, occasionally stopping to test for grit. It usually takes anywhere from 1-3 minutes, depending upon your blender.
3. In a saucepan, bring to boil 1 cup of water. Slowly add the agar while whisking. Let the pot simmer for 10 minutes, whisking as needed to ensure the agar dissolves completely. Add to the blender and mix until creamy.
4. Empty the finished mixture into an oiled container and let cool uncovered in the refrigerator.
5. When it's cooled, cover and chill for several hours.
6. To make the "Swiss holes," use a plastic straw and poke holes into the cheese at angles at random intervals.
7. Slice and enjoy on sandwiches, crackers, or any other delicious way you choose!

Fruits & Veggies

It is essential to eat plenty of fruits while you are fasting. Enjoy these according to your daily limits of net carbohydrates. This collection of keto fruits are 100 grams each for each ½ cup serving:

- Fresh Strawberries: 3 net carbs
- Raw Cranberries: 4 net carbs
- Fresh Blackberries: 5.4 net carbs
- Cantaloupe: 6 total carbs
- Fresh Blueberries: 8.2 net carbs
- Gooseberries: 8.8 net carbs
- Fresh Boysenberries: 8.8 net carbs

You need to add plenty of veggies to your lunch or dinner menu plans. Each of these has the Net Carbs listed per 100 grams or 1/2 cup serving:

- Alfalfa Seeds – Sprouted - 0.2
- Arugula – 2.05
- Asparagus - 6 spears - 2.4
- Hass Avocado - half of 1 - 1.8
- Bamboo shoots - 3
- Beans – Green snap - 3.6
- Beet greens – 0.63
- Bell pepper -2.1
- Broccoli – 4.04
- Cabbage – Savoy – 3
- Carrots – 6.78 or Baby Carrots – 5.34
- Cauliflower – 2.97
- Celery – 1.37
- Chard – 2.14
- Chicory greens – 0.7
- Chives – 1.85
- Coriander or Cilantro leaves – 0.87

- Cucumber with peel – 3.13
- Eggplant – 2.88
- Garlic – 30.96
- Ginger root – 15.77
- Kale – 5.15
- Leeks – bulb (+) lower leaf – 12.35
- Lemongrass – citronella - 25.3
- Lettuce – red leaf – 1.36
- Lettuce – ex. iceberg - 1.77
- Mushrooms brown – 3.7
- Mustard Greens – 1.47
- Onions – yellow – 7.64
- Onions – scallions or spring – 4.74
- Onions – sweet – 6.65
- Peppers – banana – 1.95
- Peppers – red hot chili – 7.31
- Peppers – jalapeno – 3.7
- Peppers – sweet – green – 2.94
- Peppers – sweet – red – 3.93
- Peppers – sweet – yellow – 5.42
- Portabella mushrooms – 2.57
- Pumpkin – 6
- Radishes – 1.8
- Seaweed – kelp – 8.27 or Seaweed – spirulina - 2.02
- Shiitake mushrooms – 4.29
- Spinach – 1.43
- Squash – crookneck - summer – 2.64
- Squash – winter – acorn – 8.92
- Tomatoes – 2.69
- Turnips – 4.63
- Turnip greens – 3.93
- Summer squash - 2.6
- Raw watercress - 3.57
- White mushrooms – 2.26
- Zucchini - 1.5

Flour Types

Almond Flour: Almond flour is a suitable replacement and is used as all-purpose flour. Each one-quarter cup portion is only three carbohydrates per gram. Step one involves blanching the almonds. Toss them into boiling water to remove the skins. Next, you will grind the flour into a finely ground product that is an excellent choice for cakes, cookies, and pie crusts. The flour has 11 grams of fat and 6 grams of carbs.

Coconut Flour: You can use coconut flour in many of the keto diet meals. When using coconut flour, remember it isn't a 1:1 ratio. In comparison, you can substitute as little as 1/3 cup to 1/4 cup of coconut flour. Use one-part water to one-part coconut flour and whisk together to use as a thickening agent. Add it to hot liquids such as soup. It's high in fiber - making it super absorbent. You can add oils, eggs, and other fluids as needed. Use coconut flour at times when you are sautéing or frying foods. The flour brings forth 4 grams of fat, 18 grams of carbs.

Sweeteners

Stevia Drops offer flavors, including English toffee, hazelnut, vanilla, and chocolate. You can make sweetened coffee or drinks quickly. However, everyone is different, and some think the drops are too bitter to taste. Therefore, only use three drops to equal one teaspoon of sugar.

The Swerve Granular Sweetener is also an excellent choice as a blend made from non-digestible carbs sourced from starchy root veggies and select fruits. It's a perfect choice for those who do not like the taste of stevia.

Swerve is on the market as a one-to-one substitute. However, start with ¾ of a teaspoon for every one of sugar. Increase the portion as needed. Swerve also has confectioners/powdered sugar for your baking needs. On the downside, it is more expensive than other products such as the Pyure.

Spices

These are a few of the popular spices used so you'll have an idea the next time you go to shake or chop (listed in grams):

- Pepper: Zero grams
- Salt: Zero – .0 grams
- Basil - 0.3 grams
- Cinnamon – .6 grams
- Garlic Powder – 1.0 grams
- Nutmeg – .6 grams
- Oregano – .1 grams
- Paprika – .4 grams
- Rosemary – .2 grams
- Thyme – .3 grams
- Dill – .4 grams

Pepper is more than pepper while you are intermittently fasting:

Black Pepper: Pepper promotes nutrient absorption in the tissues all over your body, speeds up your metabolism, and improves digestion. The main ingredient of pepper is a pipeline, which gives it a pungent taste. It can boost fat metabolism by as much as 8% for up to several hours after it's ingested. As you will see, it is used throughout your ketogenic recipes.

Cayenne Pepper: The secret ingredient in cayenne is capsaicin, a natural compound that provides the peppers with their fiery heat to provide a temporary increase in your metabolism. The peppers are also rich in vitamins, useful as an appetite controller, smooths out digestion issues, and benefit your heart health.

Italian Seasoning is used in many of your recipes. If you don't have any in your pantry; just prepare about three tablespoons using the following dry spices:

- Oregano (1 tbsp.)
- Basil (2 tsp.)
- Sage (1 tsp.)
- Thyme - not ground (2 tsp.)
- Rosemary (.5 tsp.)

Special Condiment Recipes

If you are trying to drop the pounds, and want a good substitute for mayo, try this:

Mayonnaise - Keto-Friendly

Servings Provided: 1.25 cups - 2 tbsp. each
Nutritional Content Per Serving:
- Net Carbohydrates: 0 grams
- Fat Content: 24 grams
- Protein: 1 gram
- Calories: 220

Ingredients Needed:
- Salt (.5 tsp.)
- Dry mustard (1 tsp.)
- Avocado or olive oil (1.25 cups - divided)
- Unchilled egg (1)
- Unchilled freshly squeezed lemon juice (2 tbsp.)

Preparation Technique:
1. Using a food processor, mix the mustard, salt, egg, juice, and 1/4 cup of the oil.
2. Process and slowly drizzle in the rest of the chosen oil. For the last two tablespoons - add quickly.

Chapter 5

Breakfast & Brunch Specialties

Smoothies

Almond Lover Smoothie

Servings Provided: 1
Total Preparation & Cooking Time: 5-6 minutes
Total Macro Nutrients for Each Portion:
- Net Carbs: -0- g
- Fats: 23 g
- Total Protein: 12 g
- Calorie Count: 511

Essential Ingredients:
- Almond milk (1 cup/8 oz.)
- Plain nonfat Greek yogurt (.33 cup)
- Cooked oats (.33 cup)
- Almonds (5)
- Medium banana (1)
- Almond butter (2 tbsp.)

Preparation Steps:
1. Measure all of the fixings into the cup of a NutriBullet or favorite high-speed machine.
2. Pour the milk up to the "max fill" line.
3. Blend until it is smooth and creamy.

<u>*Blueberry - Banana Bread Smoothies*</u>

Servings Provided: 2
Total Preparation & Cooking Time: 5 minutes
Total Macro Nutrients for Each Portion:
- Net Carbs: 4.7 g
- Fats: 23.3 g
- Total Protein: 3.1 g
- Calorie Count: 270

Essential Ingredients:
- Chia seeds (1 tbsp.)
- Golden flaxseed meal (3 tbsp.)
- Vanilla unsweetened coconut milk (2 cups)
- Blueberries (.25 cup)
- Liquid stevia (10 drops)
- MCT oil (2 tbsp.)
- Xanthan gum (.25 tsp.)
- Banana extract (1.5 tsp.)
- Ice cubes (2-3)

Preparation Steps:
1. Combine all of the ingredients into a blender.
2. Wait a few minutes for the seeds and flax to absorb some of the liquid.
3. Pulse for one or two minutes until well combined.
4. Add the ice to your preference.

<u>*Blueberry - Kefir Smoothies*</u>

Servings Provided: 2
Total Preparation & Cooking Time: 6-7 minutes
Total Macro Nutrients for Each Portion:
- Net Carbs: 6.6 g
- Fats: 50 g
- Total Protein: 3.9 g
- Calorie Count: 476

Essential Ingredients:
- Coconut milk kefir (1.5 cups)
- Fresh or frozen blueberries (.5 cup)
- MCT oil (2 tbsp.)
- Water (+) ice cubes (.5 cup)
- Sugar-free vanilla extract (1-2 tsp.)
  or Pure vanilla powder (.5 tsp.)

Optional Ingredients:
- Collagen powder (2 tbsp.)
- Liquid stevia/your choice (3-5 drops)

Preparation Steps:
1. Toss each of the fixings into your blender
2. Pulse until the fixings are thoroughly blended.
3. Serve in chilled glasses.

Chia Blueberry Coconut Smoothie

Servings Provided: 4
Total Preparation & Cooking Time: 4-5 minutes
Total Macro Nutrients for Each Portion:
- Net Carbs: 7.7 g
- Total Protein: 6.2 g
- Calorie Count: 249

Essential Ingredients:
- Full-fat Greek yogurt/coconut or almond milk for vegan – dairy-free (1 cup)
- Frozen blueberries (1 cup)
- Almond/cashew milk - unsweetened (1 cup)
- Ground chia seed (2 tbsp.)
- Coconut oil (2 tbsp.)
- Sweetener equivalent of sugar (2 tbsp.)
- Coconut cream (.5 cup)

- Optional: Protein powder/or another supplement

Preparation Steps:
1. Blend until all ingredients are smooth.
2. Pour into four glasses and enjoy.

Chocolate Smoothie

Servings Provided: 1 large
Total Preparation & Cooking Time: 5-6 minutes
Total Macro Nutrients for Each Portion:
- Net Carbs: 4.4 g
- Fats:46 g
- Total Protein: 34.5 g
- Calorie Count: 570

Essential Ingredients:
- Large eggs (2)
- Extra-virgin coconut oil (1 tbsp.)
- Almond/coconut butter (1-2 tbsp.)
- Coconut milk or heavy whipping cream (.25 cup)
- Chia seeds (1-2 tbsp.)
- Cinnamon (.5 tsp.)
- Stevia extract (3-5 drops)
- Plain or chocolate whey protein (.25 cup)
- Unsweetened cacao powder (1 tbsp.)
- Water (.25 cup)
- Vanilla extract (.5 tsp.)
- Ice (.5 cup)

Preparation Steps:
1. Break the eggs along with the rest of the fixings into the blender.
2. Pulse until frothy.
3. Add to a chilled glass and enjoy.

<u>*Chocolate Avocado Raspberry Smoothies – CARS*</u>

Servings Provided: 2
Total Preparation & Cooking Time: 6-7 minutes
Total Macro Nutrients for Each Portion:
- Net Carbs: 8 g
- Fats: 9.5 g
- Total Protein: 2.2 g
- Calorie Count: 133

Essential Ingredients:
- Cashew milk - ex. Silk (1.25 cups)
- Frozen raspberries (.33 cup)
- Avocado (half of 1)
- Cocoa powder (1 tbsp.)
- Raspberry extract (.125 or 1/8 tsp.)
- *Sweetener to Taste*: Powdered - ex. Swerve (1 tbsp.)

Preparation Steps:
1. Add all of the fixings into the blender
2. For a thinner smoothie, add another ¼ cup of cashew milk.

Cinnamon Roll Smoothie

Servings Provided: 1
Total Preparation & Cooking Time: 5 minutes
Total Macro Nutrients for Each Portion:
- Net Carbs: 0.6 g
- Fats: 3.3 g
- Total Protein: 26.5 g
- Calorie Count: 145

Essential Ingredients:
- Almond milk (1 cup)
- Vanilla protein powder (2 tbsp.)
- Flax meal (1 tsp.)
- Sweetener of choice (4 tsp.)
- Vanilla extract (.25 tsp.)
- Cinnamon (.5 tsp.)
- Ice (1 cup)

Preparation Steps:
1. Measure and mix each of the fixings in a blender.
2. Lastly, add the ice.
3. Mix them using the high setting for ½ minute or until it's thickened to serve.

<u>*Green Smoothie*</u>

Servings Provided: 6 @ 1 cup each
Total Preparation & Cooking Time: 5-6 minutes
Total Macro Nutrients for Each Portion:
- Net Carbs: 3 g
- Fats: 4 g
- Total Protein: 1 g
- Calorie Count: 37

Essential Ingredients:
- Romaine lettuce (1 cup)
- Freshly chopped pineapple (.33 or 1/3 cup)
- Filtered water (4 cups)
- Fresh parsley (2 tbsp.)
- Fresh ginger (1 tbsp.)
- Kiwi fruit (.5 cup)
- Raw cucumber (1 cup)
- Avocado (half of 1)
- Granulated sugar substitute - Swerve (1 tbsp.)

Preparation Steps:
1. Blend all of the ingredients until smooth.
2. You can save leftovers for several days in the refrigerator.

Mint Green Avocado Smoothie

Servings Provided: 1
Total Preparation & Cooking Time: 5 minutes
Total Macro Nutrients for Each Portion:
- Net Carbs: 5 g
- Fats: 23 g
- Total Protein: 1 g
- Calorie Count: 221

Essential Ingredients:
- Almond milk (.5 cup)
- Lime juice (1 squeeze)
- Coconut milk - full-fat (.75 cup)
- Avocado (3-4 oz./85-110 g/half of 1)
- Cilantro (3 sprigs)
- Large mint leaves (5-6)
- Vanilla extract (.25 tsp.)
- Sweetener of your choice (as desired)
- Crushed ice (1.5 cups)

Preparation Steps:
1. Measure and add all of the fixings into a blender.
2. Mix using the low-speed setting until pureed.
3. Toss in the ice and mix. Serve in a chilled glass.

Pumpkin Spice Latte Smoothie

Servings Provided: 1
Total Preparation & Cooking Time: 5-7 minutes
Total Macro Nutrients for Each Portion:
- Net Carbs: -0- g
- Fats: 3 g
- Total Protein: 4 g
- Calorie Count: 197

Essential Ingredients:
- Frozen vanilla yogurt (.33 or 1/3 cup)
- Pumpkin (.33 cup - canned ok)
- Ground cinnamon (.5 tsp.)
- Instant coffee (1 tsp.)
- Pumpkin pie spice (.5 tsp.)
- Pure maple syrup (1 tsp.)
- Greek yogurt - plain (.25 cup)
- Almond milk - unsweetened (8 oz. or 230 g)

Preparation Steps:
1. Empty all of the components into the cup of a Nutri-Bullet.
2. Pour the milk into the cup up to the 'max fill line.
3. Mix well until consistent and creamy smooth.

<u>Spinach - Cucumber Smoothies</u>

Servings Provided: 2
Total Preparation & Cooking Time: 6 minutes
Total Macro Nutrients for Each Portion:
- Net Carbs: 3 g
- Fats: 32 g
- Total Protein: 10 g
- Calorie Count: 330

Essential Ingredients:
- Ice cubes (6-7)
- Your choice of sweetener (to taste)
- Coconut milk (.75 cup)
- MCT oil (2 tbsp.)
- Cucumber (2.5 oz. or 70 g)
- Spinach (2 handfuls)
- Coconut milk (1 cup)
- Xanthan gum (.25 tsp.)

Preparation Steps:
1. Cream the coconut milk: This is a simple process. All you need to do is put the can of coconut milk in the fridge overnight. The next morning, open the can and spoon out the coconut milk that has solidified. Don't shake the can before opening it. Discard the liquids.
2. Add all of the ingredients (save the ice cubes) to a blender, and blend using the low speed until pureed. Thin with water as needed.
3. Add in the ice cubes and blend until the smoothie reaches your desired consistency.

<u>*Strawberry Smoothie*</u>

Servings Provided: 2
Total Preparation & Cooking Time: 6 minutes
Total Macro Nutrients for Each Portion:
- Net Carbs: 5.1 g
- Fats: 6.6 g
- Total Protein: 18.9 g
- Calorie Count: 156.8

Essential Ingredients:
- Large strawberries (2)
- Unsweetened almond milk (16 oz./450 g)
- Almonds (8)
- Whey protein powder (1.5 scoops)
- Cubes of ice (6)

Preparation Steps:
1. Add all of the ingredients to your blender. Wait for the ice to break apart.
2. Serve in two 10-oz./280 g chilled glasses.

Other Delicious Meals

<u>*Almond Coconut Egg Wraps*</u>

Servings Provided: 4
Total Preparation & Cooking Time: 10 minutes
Total Macro Nutrients for Each Portion:
- Net Carbs: 3 g
- Fats: 8 g
- Total Protein: 8 g
- Calorie Count: 111

Essential Ingredients:
- Organic eggs (5)
- Coconut flour (1 tbsp.)
- Sea salt (.25 tsp.)
- Almond meal (2 tbsp.)

Preparation Steps:
1. Combine the fixings in a blender and work them until creamy.
2. Heat a skillet using the med-high temperature setting.
3. Pour the batter (2 tbsp.) into the skillet. Cook - covered for three minutes.
4. Turn it over to cook for another 3 minutes.
5. Serve the wraps piping hot.

Apple Cinnamon Muffins

Servings Provided: 12
Total Preparation & Cooking Time: 25 minutes
Total Macro Nutrients for Each Portion:

- Net Carbs: 3 g
- Fats: 22 g
- Total Protein: 7 g
- Calorie Count: 241

Essential Ingredients:

- Melted ghee (.5 cup)
- Eggs (3 large)
- Almond flour (3 cups)
- Cinnamon (3 tbsp.)
- Nutmeg (1 tsp.)
- Cloves (.25 tsp.)
- Applesauce (4 tbsp.)
- Baking powder (1 tsp.)
- Lemon juice (1 tsp.)
- Stevia (as desired)

- Also Needed:
  Muffin tins (12-count - with paper or silicone cups)

Preparation Steps:

1. Program the oven setting to 350° Fahrenheit/177° Celsius.
2. Whisk the eggs and toss all of the fixings into a mixing container. Empty the batter into the prepared muffin tins.
3. Bake 17-20 minutes until the center is pushed in lightly with your fingertips and comes back quickly.

<u>*Avocado & Egg Fat Bombs with Deviled Eggs*</u>

Servings Provided: 5 @ ¾ cup each
Total Preparation & Cooking Time: 20 minutes
Total Macro Nutrients for Each Portion:
(Counts do not include egg whites and cucumber slices.)
- Net Carbs: 1.1 g
- Fats: 14.8 g
- Total Protein: 2.2 g
- Calorie Count: 147

Essential Ingredients:
- Egg yolks – cooked (3 large)
- Avocado (3.5 oz./99 g/half of 1 large)
- Keto-friendly mayonnaise (.25 cup)
- Lemon/lime juice (1 tbsp.)
- Salt – ex. Pink Himalayan (.5 tsp.)
- Chopped chives or spring onions (2 tbsp.)
- *Optional*: Fresh ground black pepper
- *Garnishes:*
  - Bell peppers
  - Lettuce Leaves
  - Cucumber slices
  - Leftover egg white halves - if using deviled eggs

Preparation Steps:
1. Prepare the eggs with salted water – 10 minutes for hard-boiled. Transfer the pot from the burner, dump, and add cold water.
2. Remove the shells when cooled. Slice them into halves, and remove the yolks into a bowl without breaking the whites.
3. Peel and remove the seeds from the avocado. Chop and load the processor with avocado, mayonnaise, egg yolks, salt, lemon juice, and pepper if desired.
4. Add the creamy mixture to the egg halves or cucumber slices.
5. Pop them into the refrigerator in a closed container for up to five days.

<u>*Bacon & Avocado Omelet*</u>

Servings Provided: 1
Total Preparation & Cooking Time: 40 minutes
Total Macro Nutrients for Each Portion:
- Net Carbs: 3.3 g
- Fats: 63 g
- Total Protein: 30 g
- Calorie Count: 719

Essential Ingredients:
- Crispy bacon (1 slice)
- Large organic eggs (2)
- Freshly grated parmesan cheese (.5 cup)
- Ghee or coconut oil or butter (2 tbsp.)
- Avocado (half of 1 small)

Preparation Steps:
1. Prepare the bacon to your liking and set aside.
2. Combine the eggs, parmesan cheese, and your choice of finely chopped herbs.
3. Warm a skillet and add the butter/ghee to melt using the med-high temperature setting.
4. After the pan is heated, whisk and add the eggs.
5. Prepare the omelet working it towards the middle of the pan for about 30 seconds. When firm, flip, and cook it for another 30 seconds.
6. Arrange the omelet on a plate and garnish it with the crunched bacon bits. Serve with sliced avocado.

<u>*Baked Apples*</u>

Servings Provided: 4
Total Preparation & Cooking Time: 1 hour 15 minutes
Total Macro Nutrients for Each Portion:
- Net Carbs: 16 g
- Fats: 19.9 g
- Total Protein: 6.8 g
- Calorie Count: 175

Essential Ingredients:
- Keto-friendly sweetener (4 tsp. or to taste)
- Cinnamon (.75 tsp.)
- Chopped pecans (.25 cup)
- Granny Smith apples (4 large)

Preparation Steps:
1. Set the oven temperature at 375° Fahrenheit/191° Celsius.
2. Mix the sweetener with cinnamon and pecans.
3. Core the apple and add the prepared stuffing.
4. Add enough water into the baking dish to cover the bottom of the apple.
5. Bake them for about 45 minutes to 1 hour.

Blueberry Muffins

Servings Provided: 12
Total Preparation & Cooking Time: 55 minutes
Total Macro Nutrients for Each Portion:
- Net Carbs: 5 g
- Fats: 20 g
- Total Protein: 6 g
- Calorie Count: 221

Essential Ingredients:
- Almond flour (2 cups or 224 g)
- Coconut flour (.25 cup or 30 g)
- Baking powder (4 g or 1 tsp.)
- Konjac root fiber (2 tsp. or 8 g)
- Baking soda (4 g or 1 tsp.)
- Salt (1 pinch)
- Olive oil (.5 cup or 108 g)
- Fresh eggs (3 large or 150 g)
- Water (2-4 tbsp.)
- Fresh blueberries (.5 cup or 74 g)

Preparation Steps:
1. Set the oven temperature at 350° Fahrenheit/177° Celsius.
2. Cover the muffin tin with 12 paper/foil liners.
3. Whisk/sift the almond flour with coconut flour, baking powder, salt, konjac root fiber, and baking soda.
4. Mix in the eggs with olive oil and two tablespoons of water into the dry components. Thoroughly whisk to combine (as the consistency of thick pancake batter).
5. Gently fold in the blueberries (about half to two-thirds full).
6. Bake the muffins until a toothpick inserted into the center remains clean when removed (35-40 min.). Serve when ready.

<u>*Breakfast Skillet*</u>

Servings Provided: 2
Total Preparation & Cooking Time: 20-25 minutes
Total Macro Nutrients for Each Portion:
- Net Carbs: 7.1 g
- Fats: 32 g
- Total Protein: 65.2 g
- Calorie Count: 556

Essential Ingredients:
- Organic ground turkey/grass-fed beef (.75 to 1 lb./340-450 g)
- Organic eggs (6)
- Keto-friendly salsa of choice (1 cup)

Preparation Steps:
1. Warm the oil in a skillet using a medium-temperature setting. Add the turkey and cook till the pink is gone.
2. Fold in the salsa and simmer for two to three minutes.
3. Crack the eggs over the turkey base. Put a top on the pot and cook for seven minutes until the egg whites are opaque as desired.

Servings Provided: 4
Total Preparation & Cooking Time: 25-30 minutes
Total Macro Nutrients for Each Portion:
- Net Carbs: 6 g
- Fats: 48 g
- Total Protein: 18 g
- Calorie Count: 527

Essential Ingredients:
- Eggs (4)
- Butter (5 tbsp./divided into 2 + 3 tbsp.)
- Cayenne pepper (.25 tsp.)
- Salt (.5 tsp.)
- Olive oil (1 tbsp.)
- Sour cream (.5 cup)
- Lemon juice (2 tbsp.)
- Asparagus (24 oz./680 g)
- Parmesan cheese - grated (3 oz./85 g)

Preparation Steps:
1. Thoroughly cook the eggs in two tablespoons of the butter over medium heat until they are set - not dry.
2. Pour the cooked eggs into a blender while they are still hot, and add the pepper, salt, sour cream, and parmesan cheese. Blend using the low-speed setting until this mix is creamy and smooth.
3. Fry the asparagus in a skillet using a low-temperature setting in olive oil for five minutes.
4. Then add the three tablespoons of butter to the skillet and let it melt completely.
5. Turn off the burner and pour in the blended egg mixture with the lemon juice and let it thoroughly set.
6. After ten minutes, return the pan to heat, add in the asparagus, and stir to mix thoroughly. Place all items on a plate and serve.

Servings Provided: 6
Total Preparation & Cooking Time: 25 minutes
Total Macro Nutrients for Each Portion:
- Net Carbs: 1 g
- Fats: 7 g
- Total Protein: 8 g
- Calorie Count: 101

Essential Ingredients:
- Bacon (6 strips)
- Large eggs (6)
- Cheese (.25 cup)
- Fresh spinach (1 handful)
- Pepper & Salt (as desired)

Preparation Steps:
1. Set the oven setting to 400° Fahrenheit/204° Celsius.
2. Prepare the bacon using medium heat on the stovetop. Place on towels to drain.
3. Grease six muffin tins with a spritz of oil. Line each muffin tin with a bacon slice, pressing tightly to make a secure well for the eggs.
4. Drain and dry the spinach with a paper towel. Whisk the eggs and combine them with the spinach.
5. Add the mixture to the prepared tins and sprinkle with cheese. Sprinkle with pepper and salt until it is like you like it.
6. Bake for 15 minutes. Remove when done and serve or cool to store in the fridge.

<u>Flaxseed Porridge</u>

Servings Provided: 1
Total Preparation & Cooking Time: 5 minutes
Total Macro Nutrients for Each Portion:
- Net Carbs: 4 g
- Fats: 40 g
- Total Protein: 6 g

Essential Ingredients:
- Flaxseed - plain or roasted is nutty-like (3 tbsp.)
- Coconut Milk - unsweetened (.5 cup)
- Butter (2.5 tsp.)
- Grapeseed oil (2 tsp.)
- Wild/frozen blueberries (2 tbsp.)
- Cinnamon (.125 tsp.)

Preparation Steps:
1. Whisk the milk with the flaxseed in a microwave-safe bowl. Use one that will hold at least two cups of liquid. Cook until the mixture starts rising (30-45 sec.).
2. Transfer the container to the countertop and wait for it to cool for one minute.
3. Mix in the butter, oil, blueberries, and cinnamon. Stir thoroughly to coat the blueberries. Don't over-stir; it will make the porridge gummy. *Note:* You can also make it using a small saucepan on the stovetop. You will remove the pan from the burner once the mixture starts to boil.

Chapter 6

Lunchtime & Dinner Soup
& Salad Favorites

Soup Options

Broccoli "N" Cheese Soup - Crock Pot

Servings Provided: 3
Total Preparation & Cooking Time: 4 hours 10 minutes
Total Macro Nutrients for Each Portion:
- Net Carbohydrates: 6.6 g
- Fats: 21.4 g
- Total Protein: 3.5 g
- Calorie Count: 215

Essential Ingredients:
- Vegetable broth (1 cup)
- Coconut cream (.5 cup)
- Broccoli (1 cup)
- Cheddar cheese (1 cup)

Preparation Steps:
1. Add each of the ingredients into a crockpot. After breakfast, just turn on the pot, and you will be ready for lunch.
2. Set the timer for four hours using the low-temperature setting.
3. Serve it piping hot.

Buffalo Chicken Soup

Servings Provided: 6
Total Preparation & Cooking Time: 45 minutes
Total Macro Nutrients for Each Portion:
- Net Carbs: 4 g
- Fats: 17 g
- Total Protein: 33 g
- Calorie Count: 335

Essential Ingredients:
- Olive oil (1 tbsp.)
- Medium onion (1)
- Chopped celery (2 cups)
- Dried thyme (1 tsp.)
- Chicken breasts (4)
- Hot sauce - ex. - Frank's Red (.25 cup/as desired)
- Chicken stock (4 cups)
- Garlic powder (1 tsp.)
- Cream cheese (4 oz./110 g)
- Crumbled blue cheese (.5 cup + more for serving)

Preparation Steps:
1. Dice the celery and onion.
2. Set the Instant Pot using the sauté mode to warm the oil. Dice/chop and add the celery and onions. Sauté them until they're starting to soften.
3. Measure and shake in the garlic powder and thyme. Sauté the mixture for a couple of minutes.
4. Meanwhile, trim the chicken and remove the skin and bones. Slice it into lengthwise strips.
5. Toss the chicken, hot sauce, and chicken stock into the cooker.
6. Securely close the lid and set the timer for 15 minutes using the high-pressure setting.
7. At that time, natural-release the pressure for ten minutes.

Next, quick-release the remainder of the built-up steam.

8. Dice the cream cheese into chunks and crumble the blue cheese.
9. Transfer the chicken to a cutting block to dice/shred it into chunks.
10. Next, mix in both varieties of cheese to the hot soup.
11. Whisk the soup and add the shredded chicken back into the pot.
12. Serve it hot with the blue cheese and hot sauce to your liking.

Cabbage Roll 'Unstuffed' Soup

Servings Provided: 9
Total Preparation & Cooking Time: 25 minutes
Total Macro Nutrients for Each Portion:
- Net Carbs: 3 g
- Fats: 15 g
- Total Protein: 16 g
- Calorie Count: 217

Essential Ingredients:
- Minced garlic cloves (2)
- Small diced onion (half of 1)
- 80/20 Ground beef (1.5 lb./680 g)
- Bragg's Aminos (.25 cup)
- Tomato sauce (8 oz./230 g can)
- Beef broth (3 cups)
- Keto-friendly Worcestershire sauce/another substitute (3 tsp.)
- Diced tomatoes (14 oz./400 g can)
- Chopped cabbage (1 medium)
- Pepper and salt (.5 tsp. each)
- Parsley (.5 tsp.)
- _Also Needed:_ Instant Pot

Preparation Steps:
1. Prepare using the sauté function on the Instant Pot to brown the beef, garlic, and onions.
2. Drain and add the mixture into the cooker with the remainder of the fixings.
3. Program the unit on the soup function.
4. Natural-release the soup for about ten minutes, and quick-release the rest of the steam. Stir and serve.

Cauliflower & Kielbasa Soup

Servings Provided: 4
Total Preparation & Cooking Time: 40 minutes
Total Macro Nutrients for Each Portion:
- Net Carbs: 5.7 g
- Fats: 19 g
- Total Protein: 10 g
- Calorie Count: 251

Essential Ingredients:
- Ghee (3 tbsp.)
- Cauliflower (1 head)
- Rutabaga (1)
- Kielbasa sausage (1)
- Chicken broth (2 cups)
- Small onion (1)
- Water (2 cups)
- Black pepper and salt (as desired)

Preparation Steps:
1. Chop the cauliflower, onions, and rutabaga. Slice the sausage.
2. Melt two tablespoons of the ghee in a soup pot. Sauté it for three minutes.
3. Toss in the rutabaga and cauliflower. Sauté it for about five minutes.
4. Pour in the water, broth, pepper, and salt. Boil for about 20 minutes.
5. Melt the butter in a skillet to cook the sausage (5 min.).
6. Puree the soup until it's smooth and serve with the kielbasa.

Servings Provided: 6
Total Preparation & Cooking Time: 6 hours 40 minutes
Total Macro Nutrients for Each Portion:
- Net Carbs: 3 g
- Fats: 31.4 g
- Total Protein: 23 g
- Calorie Count: 425

Essential Ingredients:
- Chicken breasts (1.5 lb./680 g)
- Mixed vegetables (preferably broccoli & cauliflower (6 cups)
- Full fat coconut milk (1 can)
- Crushed tomatoes (1 cup)
- Ground coriander (2 tsp.)
- Cumin (1 tbsp.)
- Ground ginger (2 tsp.)
- Cinnamon (1 tsp.)
- Ground ginger powder (2 tsp.)
- Cayenne pepper (.5 tsp.)
- Water (1 cup)
- Salt (to taste)

Preparation Steps:
1. Trim the chicken, removing all fat and bones. Toss the chicken and vegetables in the Crockpot.
2. Mix in the remainder of the fixings - stir to mix everything.
3. Close the lid and cook on low for six hours. Serve when it's ready.

<u>Chili Delight - No-Beans - Stovetop</u>

Servings Provided: 6
Total Preparation & Cooking Time: 2 hours 15 minutes
Total Macro Nutrients for Each Portion:
- Net Carbs: 5 g
- Fats: 14 g
- Total Protein: 26 g
- Calorie Count: 263

Essential Ingredients:
- Water (3 cups)
- Ground beef 1.5 lb./680 g)
- Cumin (.75 tsp.)
- Black pepper (.75 tsp.)
- Cinnamon (.25 tsp.)
- Garlic cloves (2)
- Chopped onion (.25 cup)
- Worcestershire sauce (1 tsp.)
- Bay leaves (3)
- Salt (1.5 tsp.)
- Allspice (.5 tsp.)
- Chili powder (2 tbsp.)
- Red pepper (.5 tsp.)
- Tomato paste (170 g/6 oz.)
- Sliced black olives (2.25 oz./63 g)
- Finely chopped chili peppers (.25 cup)

Preparation Steps:
1. Break apart the ground beef in a large stew pot on the stovetop. Drain away the juices.
2. Mince the garlic. Combine with the rest of the fixings. Wait for the mixture to boil. Simmer the chili for two hours to serve.

<u>Creamy Chicken Soup</u>

Servings Provided: 4
Total Preparation & Cooking Time: 10-15 minutes
Total Macro Nutrients for Each Portion:
- Net Carbs: 2 g
- Fats: 25 g
- Total Protein: 18 g
- Calorie Count: 307

Essential Ingredients:
- Butter (2 tbsp.)
- Large breast of chicken (1-2 cups - shredded)
- Cubed cream cheese (4 oz./110 g)
- Garlic seasoning (2 tbsp.)
- Chicken broth (14.5 oz./410 g)
- Salt (to taste)
- Heavy cream (.25 cup)

Preparation Steps:
1. Heat a saucepan. Melt the butter using the medium temperature setting.
2. Mix in the shredded chicken and toss with the cream cheese and seasoning.
3. When it is all melted, stir in the heavy cream and broth.
4. Once it's boiling, adjust the temperature setting. Simmer for three to four minutes.
5. Season the soup as desired before serving.

Mexican Chicken Soup

Servings Provided: 6
Total Preparation & Cooking Time: varies - 6-8 hours
Total Macro Nutrients for Each Portion:
- Net Carbs: 5 g
- Fats: 23 g
- Total Protein: 28 g
- Calorie Count: 400

Essential Ingredients:
- Chicken thighs (1.5 lb. or 680 g)
- Chicken broth (15 oz. or 430 g)
- Pepper Jack/Monterey cheese (8 oz. or 230 g)
- Chunky salsa – ex. Tostitos (15.5 oz. or 440 g)
- Also Needed: Slow Cooker

Preparation Steps:
1. Cut out any bones and remove the fat from the chicken. Arrange them in the slow cooker.
2. Mix in the rest of the fixings. Prepare using the low setting (6-8 hrs.) or the high setting (3 to 4 hrs.).
3. When the time is up, remove and shred the chicken. Put it back in the cooker to mingle with the juices for a minute or so.
4. Stir and serve - right out of the cooker.

Salad Options

Avocado Shrimp Salad

Servings Provided: 4
Total Preparation & Cooking Time: 20 minutes
Total Macro Nutrients for Each Portion:
- Net Carbs: 4 g
- Fats: 13 g
- Total Protein: 27 g
- Calorie Count: 255

Essential Ingredients:
- Shrimp (1 lb. - small-size - 450 g)
- Olive oil (1 tsp.)
- Lime juice (.25 cup)
- Cilantro - fresh (2 tbsp.)
- Salt & black pepper (1 tsp. each)
- Red onion (.25 cup)
- Tomato (1 small)
- Avocado (1)

Preparation Steps:
1. Cook, peel, and devein the shrimp.
2. Dice the tomato and onion.
3. Peel, pit, and dice the avocado.
4. Mix the lime juice with the oil, pepper, and salt in a medium-sized mixing container.
5. Chop and add in the cilantro, avocado, tomato, red onion, and shrimp and thoroughly mix.

Chicken & Bacon Chopped Salad

Servings Provided: 6
Total Preparation & Cooking Time: 20 minutes
Total Macro Nutrients for Each Portion:
Dressing @ 2 tbsp. + salad @ 2.33 cups:
- Net Carbs: 2 g
- Fats: 22 g
- Total Protein: 35 g
- Calorie Count: 348

Essential Ingredients:
- Frozen grilled chicken breast strips (22 oz./620 g pkg.)
- Crumbled blue cheese (1 cup)
- White wine vinegar (3 tbsp.)
- Coarsely ground pepper (.125 or 1/8 tsp.)
- Water (1 tbsp.)
- Canola oil (.25 cup)
- Chopped romaine (8 cups)
- Tomatoes (3 medium)
- Bacon strips (6 cooked & crumbled)

Preparation Steps:
1. Heat chicken according to package directions. Cool slightly; coarsely chop chicken. Cook and crumble the bacon.
2. Make the dressing by combining the cheese, vinegar, water, and pepper in a small food processor, processing until creamy. Gradually add in the oil in a steady stream.
3. Chop the tomatoes. In a large bowl, combine romaine, chicken, tomatoes, and bacon.
4. Serve with dressing.

<u>Chicken Caesar Salad with Avocado & Bacon</u>

Servings Provided: 2
Total Preparation & Cooking Time: 5-10 minutes
Total Macro Nutrients for Each Portion:
- Net Carbs: 3 g
- Fats: 27 g
- Total Protein: 19 g
- Calorie Count: 337

Essential Ingredients:
- Grilled – pre-cooked chicken breast (1)
- Ripe sliced avocado (1)
- Crumbled bacon (1 cup)
- Marie's Creamy Caesar Dressing/your preference (6 tbsp.)

Preparation Steps:
1. Slice the chicken and avocado into one-inch slices.
2. Combine the ingredients and add the dressing (3 tbsp. each).

<u>*Cheesy Salad Sandwich*</u>

Servings Provided: 1
Total Preparation & Cooking Time: 6-7 minutes
Total Macro Nutrients for Each Portion:
- Net Carbs: 4.5 g
- Fats: 15 g
- Total Protein: 4 g
- Calorie Count: 104

Essential Ingredients:
- Butter (.5 oz./14 g)
- Romaine or baby gem lettuce (2 oz./56 g)
- Edam cheese (1 oz./28 g)
- Cherry tomato (1 sliced)
- Sliced avocado (half of 1)

Preparation Steps:
1. Rinse the lettuce and slice the rest of the ingredients.
2. Add butter on the leaves with a layer of cheese, avocado, and tomato. Top it off with lettuce and serve.

Crunchy Cauliflower & Pine Nut Salad

Servings Provided: 1
Total Preparation & Cooking Time: 2.5 hours
Total Macro Nutrients for Each Portion:
- Net Carbs: 8 g
- Fats: 63 g
- Total Protein: 10 g
- Calorie Count: 638

Essential Ingredients:
- Cauliflower (.25 cup)
- Leeks/onion (2 tbsp.)
- Pine nuts (.25 cup)
- Sour cream (2 tbsp.)
- Iceberg lettuce (.5 cup)
- Mayonnaise (.25 cup)
- Feta cheese (.25 cup)

Preparation Steps:
1. Chop the cauliflower, onion, and pine nuts. Shred the lettuce.
2. Toast the pine nuts using the medium-temperature setting.
3. Mix each of the fixings in a big mixing container - place them in the fridge for a minimum of two hours.
4. Serve cold.

Grab & Go Jar Salad

Yields Provided: 1
Total Preparation & Cooking Time: 20 minutes
Nutritional Facts Per Serving:
- Net Carbohydrates: 4 grams
- Fat Content: 19 grams
- Protein: 8 grams
- Calories: 215

Essential Ingredients:
- Black pepper & salt (as desired)
- Keto-friendly mayonnaise (4 tbsp.)
- Scallion (.5)
- Cucumber (.25 oz. or 7 g)
- Red bell pepper (.25 oz. or 7 g)
- Cherry tomatoes (.25 oz. or 7 g)
- Leafy greens (.25 oz. or 7 g)
- Seasoned tempeh (4 oz. or 110 g)

Preparation Steps:
1. Chop or shred the vegetables as desired.
2. Layer in the dark leafy greens first, followed by the onions, tomato, bell peppers, avocado, and shredded carrot.
3. Top with the tempeh, or use the same amount of another high-protein option to mix things up in later weeks.
4. Top with keto-vegan mayonnaise before serving.

<u>*Greek Chopped Salad*</u>

Servings Provided: 2
Total Preparation & Cooking Time: 10 minutes
Total Macro Nutrients for Each Portion:
- Net Carbs: 2 g
- Fats: 4 g
- Total Protein: 4 g
- Calorie Count: 202

Essential Ingredients:
- Chopped romaine (2 cups)
- Halved grape tomatoes (.5 cup)
- Kalamata black olives (.25 cup)
- Crumbled feta cheese (.25 cup)
- Olive oil (1 tbsp.)
- Vinaigrette dressing (2 tbsp.)
- Black pepper & Pink salt (as desired)

Preparation Steps:
1. Put the salad together using lettuce as a base.
2. Spritz it using a drizzle of oil and vinegar.
3. Serve in two salad dishes.

Servings Provided: 6
Total Preparation & Cooking Time: 20 minutes
Total Macro Nutrients for Each Portion:
- Net Carbs: 4 g
- Fats: 9 g
- Total Protein: 24 g
- Calorie Count: 209

Essential Ingredients:
- Ripe avocados (2 medium)
- Cooked shrimp (1.5 lb./680 g @ 31-40 per lb.)
- Pico de gallo (1 cup)
- Clamato juice (.5 cup - chilled)
- Lime juice (2 tbsp.)
- Kosher salt (.25 tsp.)
- Ground cumin (.25 tsp.)
- Hot pepper sauce (.25 tsp./less if desired)
- Black pepper (1 dash)
- _Optional_: Lime wedges

Preparation Steps:
1. Peel and slice the avocado into ½-inch pieces. Peel, devein the shrimp and remove the tails.
2. Toss all of the fixings into a large mixing container.
3. Divide the salad into serving dishes and enjoy them!

<u>Steak Salad</u>

Servings Provided: 2
Total Preparation & Cooking Time: 20 minutes
Total Macro Nutrients for Each Portion:
- Net Carbs: 1.5 g
- Fats: 33 g
- Total Protein: 1.5 g
- Calorie Count: 403

Essential Ingredients:
- Steakhouse seasoning (1 tbsp.)
- Pepper and salt (to taste)
- Ribeye steak (1 @ 8 oz./230 g)
- Green salad mix (2 cups)
- Olive oil (1 tbsp.)
- Wine vinegar (1 tsp.)

Preparation Steps:
1. Use the steak seasoning to prepare the steak and cook as desired.
2. Wait for it to cool while you toss the salad fixings with a dusting of pepper and salt.
3. Drizzle with oil and toss again.
4. Slice the steak into bite-sized strips.
5. Arrange the salad on two serving dishes and sprinkle the steak bits on top.
6. Serve using your favorite dressing if desired - but count the carbs.

<u>*Vegetarian Club Salad*</u>

Servings Provided:
Total Preparation & Cooking Time: 10 minutes
Total Macro Nutrients for Each Portion:
- Net Carbs: 5 g
- Fats: 27 g
- Total Protein: 17 g
- Calorie Count: 330

Essential Ingredients:
- Dijon mustard (1 tbsp.)
- Parsley - dried (1 tsp.)
- Onion powder (.5 tsp.)
- Garlic powder (.5 tsp.)
- Cucumber - diced (1 cup)
- Cherry tomatoes (.5 cup) cut in half
- Romaine lettuce (3 cups) cut into pieces
- Mayonnaise (2 tbsp.)
- Sour cream (2 tbsp.)
- Swiss cheese - cubed (1 cup)
- Eggs - hard-boiled (3 sliced)

Preparation Steps:
1. Mix the sour cream, mayonnaise, and herbs until mixed well to make the salad dressing.
2. Prepare the salads in three bowls by mixing in layers the cheese cubes, sliced eggs, and the fresh vegetables.
3. Drop one teaspoon of Dijon mustard in the center of each salad. Serve with the already prepared dressing on the side.

Pasta Favorites

Asian BBQ Meatball Noodle Bowl

Servings Provided: 4
Total Preparation & Cooking Time: 20-25 minutes
Total Macro Nutrients for Each Portion:
- Net Carbs: 10.5 g
- Fats: 19.7 g
- Total Protein: 23.6 g
- Calorie Count: 318

Essential Ingredients:
The Meatballs:
- Ground chicken or turkey (1 lb./450 g)
- Shiitake mushrooms (.25 cup)
- Fresh cilantro (.25 cup)
- Green onions (2)
- Garlic cloves (2)
- Tamari (1 tbsp.)
- Fish sauce (1 tsp.)
- Salt (.5 tsp.)
- Red pepper flakes (.5 tsp.)
- Sesame oil (2 tbsp.)

The BBQ Sauce:
- Sesame oil (1 tbsp.)
- Rice wine vinegar (.25 cup)
- Tamari (.25 cup)
- Granulated swerve (.25 cup)
- Sriracha (3 tbsp.)
- Fresh ginger (1 tbsp.)
- Clove of garlic (1)

Other Fixings:
- Snow peas (8 oz./230 g)
- Shirataki/Miracle noodles (2 pkg.)

Preparation Steps:
1. Mince the mushrooms, onions, ginger, and garlic.
2. Combine all of the meatball fixings (omitting the oil). Roll into 16 balls.
3. Whisk the sauce fixings and noodles. Set both aside for now.
4. Meanwhile, warm the oil in the skillet and add the meatballs - single layered.
5. Sear for 2-3 minutes on each side and remove from the heat.
6. Add the peas to the skillet to simmer for one minute until it starts to wilt.
7. Arrange the meatballs in the mixture and stir.
8. Simmer with a lid on the pot for about three minutes.

Servings Provided: 2
Total Preparation & Cooking Time: 40-45 minutes
Total Macro Nutrients for Each Portion:
- Net Carbs: 10.5 g
- Fats: 29.5 g
- Total Protein: 18.5 g
- Calorie Count: 397

Essential Ingredients:
- Butternut squash or pumpkin (1 cup)
- Cauliflower (2 cups)
- Diced organic bacon (1-1.5 cups)
- Zoodles - zucchini noodles (3 cups)
- Turmeric (.25 to .5 tbsp.)
- Salt (to taste)
- Grass-fed butter or ghee (2-3 tbsp.)
- Filtered water/chicken bone broth (.25 cup)
- Fresh sage leaves (1 handful)

Preparation Steps:
1. Steam the pumpkin and cauliflower in a saucepan until softened. Dice and toss the bacon into a skillet and fry until crispy.
2. Remove the bacon from the skillet when it's crispy, and place it on a paper-lined dish to drain. Leave the fat in the frying pan.
3. Sauté the sage leaves in the bacon fat/grease until browned and crispy. Transfer the leaves to the plate with the bacon.
4. Toss the zoodles into a saucepan and steam for a few minutes.
5. Combine the cauliflower, butter/ghee, cooked squash/pumpkin, turmeric, salt, and two tablespoons of the broth into a food processor. Pulse until smooth and creamy. Continue adding water by the spoonful to reach the desired sauce consistency.
6. When the zoodles are ready, place them onto two serving platters.

7. Pour the creamy sauce on top, adding a sprinkle of the bacon pieces and crispy sage leaves.
8. Serve immediately.

Baked Zucchini Noodles With Feta

Servings Provided: 3
Total Preparation & Cooking Time: 25 minutes
Total Macro Nutrients for Each Portion:
- Net Carbs: 5 g
- Fats: 8 g
- Total Protein: 4 g
- Calorie Count: 105

Essential Ingredients:
- Spiralized zucchini (2)
- Quartered plum tomato (1)
- Feta cheese (8 cubes)
- Pepper and salt (1 tsp. each)
- Olive oil (1 tbsp.)

Preparation Steps:
1. Lightly grease a roasting pan with a spritz of cooking oil.
2. Set the oven temperature at 375° Fahrenheit/191° Celsius.
3. Slice the noodles with a spiralizer, and add the olive oil, tomatoes, pepper, and salt.
4. Bake the noodle dish for 10 to 15 minutes. Transfer from the oven and add the cheese cubes, tossing to combine. Serve.

Servings Provided: 6
Total Preparation & Cooking Time: 20 minutes
Total Macro Nutrients for Each Portion:
- Net Carbs: 5.1 g
- Fats: 14.2 g
- Total Protein: 17.4 g
- Calorie Count: 232.8

Essential Ingredients:
- Olive oil (2 tbsp.)
- Salmon fillets (4 @ 4 oz./110 g each)
- Carrot (1 small)
- Orange bell pepper (1 medium)
- Shallot (2 tbsp.)
- Sesame oil (2 tbsp.)
- Japanese 7-Spice Shichimi - shichimi togarashi (2 tbsp.)
- Liquid Aminos/Soy sauce alternative of choice (4 tbsp.)
- Riced cauliflower (1 medium)
- Pepper & salt (as desired)

Preparation Steps:
1. Cube the salmon into two-inch pieces. Chop the peppers and carrots and finely dice the shallot. Prepare the cauliflower.
2. Preheat a stockpot with oil using the medium-temperature setting. Add and sauté the salmon for about five minutes until they turn white.
3. Toss in the shallots, peppers, and carrots – continue sautéing for another five minutes.
4. Mix in the sesame oil and aminos to coat the fish and veggies. Sprinkle in the 7-spice powder and let it rest for two to three minutes.
5. Toss in the cauliflower and mix with a wooden spoon. Raise the temperature setting to med-high. Fry the cauliflower,

stirring occasionally.
6. Flavor with pepper and salt if desired.

Chapter 7

Lunchtime
& Dinner Poultry Specialties

Balsamic Chicken Thighs - Slow Cooker

Servings Provided: 8
Total Preparation & Cooking Time: 4 hours 10-15 minutes
Total Macro Nutrients for Each Portion:
- Net Carbs: 3.6 g
- Fats: 4 g
- Total Protein: 20.1 g
- Calorie Count: 133

Essential Ingredients:
- Chicken thighs (8/24 oz. approx.)
- Garlic (4 cloves)
- Dried minced onion (2 tsp.)
- EVOO (1 tbsp.)
- Garlic powder (1 tsp.)
- Dried basil (1 tsp.)
- Pepper and salt (.5 tsp. each)
- Balsamic vinegar (.5 cup)
- Parsley (as desired)

Preparation Steps:
1. Trim the chicken - removing all of the bones. Mince the garlic and chop the parsley.
2. Mix all of the dry spices (minced onion, pepper, salt, basil, and garlic powder). Rub over the chicken and set it aside for now.

3. Pour the extra-virgin olive oil and garlic into the slow cooker and add the chicken.
4. Empty the vinegar over the thighs and place the lid.
5. Cook for four hours using the high-temperature setting.
6. Sprinkle with the freshly chopped parsley, serve, and enjoy.

<u>*BBQ Chicken Casserole*</u>

Servings Provided: 8
Total Preparation & Cooking Time: 45 minutes
Total Macro Nutrients for Each Portion:
- Net Carbs: 4 g
- Fats: 44 g
- Total Protein: 41.5 g
- Calorie Count: 601.5

Essential Ingredients:
- Cooked chicken breast/thighs (2 lb. or 910 g)
- Cooked bacon (8 oz. or 230 g)
- Frozen chopped spinach (230 g/8 oz.)
- Keto bbq sauce (.75 cup)
- Keto ranch dressing (2/3 cup)
- Unchilled cream cheese (8 oz. or 230 g)
- Hot smoked paprika (1 tsp.)
- Black pepper (.25 tsp.)
- Sea salt (.5 tsp.)
- Sharp cheddar cheese (2 cups)
- Also Needed: 9 x 9 or 23 x 3-cm baking dish

Preparation Steps:
1. Warm the oven to reach 350° Fahrenheit/177° Celsius.
2. Do the prep. Thaw the spinach. Cook the bacon and shred the chicken (cooking times not in total counts).
3. Shred the chicken, crush the bacon and spinach in a big salad container.
4. Use a food processor or stand mixer to mix the bbq sauce with the ranch dressing, cream cheese, salt, pepper, and smoked paprika. Process until smooth.
5. Toss the chicken mixture with the bbq sauce mixture and transfer the mixture into the baking dish.
6. Garnish it using cheese and bake the casserole for ½ hour to serve.

<u>*Buffalo Wings*</u>

Servings Provided: 2
Total Preparation & Cooking Time: 30 minutes
Total Macro Nutrients for Each Portion:
- Net Carbs: 1 g
- Fats: 46 g
- Total Protein: 48 g
- Calorie Count: 620

Essential Ingredients:
- Chicken drumettes/wingettes/wings (6)
- Butter (2 tbsp.)
- Red hot sauce (.5 cup)
    To Taste:
- Pepper & salt
- Garlic powder
- Paprika
- *Optional*: Cayenne pepper

Preparation Steps:
1. Break the wings apart, removing the tips to make the wing drumettes.
2. Pour the sauce over the wings, and add the spices.
3. It is best to let the pan sit in the fridge for an hour if you have time.
4. Set the broiler on the high setting and arrange the rack six inches from the chicken wings—Cook for eight minutes. Flip them and cook for another six to eight minutes.
5. In a pot, melt the butter and the remainder of the hot sauce.
6. Transfer the pan to a cool burner and mix in the sauce - toss to cover them using the sauce.

<u>*Cheesy Bacon Chicken*</u>

Servings Provided: 6
Total Preparation & Cooking Time: 55-60 minutes
Total Macro Nutrients for Each Portion:
- Net Carbs: 1 g
- Fats: 23 g
- Total Protein: 29 g
- Calorie Count: 345

Essential Ingredients:
- Chicken breasts - cut in half widthwise (2.5 to 3 lbs./1.1 to 1.4-kg./5 to 6 pieces)
- Seasoning rub/seasoning salt or a mix of salt, garlic powder, onion powder, paprika (2 tbsp.)
- Bacon - cut strips in half (.5 lb./230 g)
- Shredded cheddar (4 oz./110 g)
- Sugar-free barbecue sauce - optional for serving

Preparation Steps:
1. Warm the oven to reach 400° Fahrenheit/204° Celsius.
2. Spray a large rimmed baking sheet with cooking spray.
3. Rub both sides of chicken breasts with seasoning rub.
4. Top each with a piece of bacon. Bake for ½ hour on the top rack until the chicken is 160° Fahrenheit/71° Celsius and the bacon looks crispy.
5. Transfer the pan to the countertop and sprinkle the cheese over the bacon.
6. Bake it for another ten minutes or until the cheese is bubbly and golden.
7. Serve with barbecue sauce.

<u>Chicken Parmesan</u>

Servings Provided: 2
Total Preparation & Cooking Time: 50 minutes
Total Macro Nutrients for Each Portion:
Net Carbs: 3 g
Fats: 32 g
Total Protein: 74 g
Calorie Count: 600

Essential Ingredients:
- Chicken breasts (450 g/1 lb.)
- Parmesan cheese (2 tbsp.)
- Pork rinds (1 oz./28 g)
- Egg (1)
- Marinara sauce (.5 cup)
- Shredded mozzarella (.5 cup)

To Your Liking:
- Pepper and salt
- Oregano
- Garlic powder

Preparation Steps:
1. Set the oven temperature to 350° Fahrenheit/177° Celsius.
2. Lightly grease a baking tray using a misting of cooking oil spray.
3. Use a food processor/Magic Bullet to crush the pork rinds and parmesan cheese. Add them to a bowl.
4. Pound the chicken breasts until they are ½-inch thick. Beat the egg, and dip the chicken in for an egg wash. Dip the chicken into the crumbs.
5. Arrange the breasts in the prepared pan - dust with the seasonings.
6. Set a timer to bake for 25 minutes. Empty the marinara sauce over each breast portion. Top with the mozzarella and bake for another 15 minutes.
7. Enjoy with some spaghetti squash or a bed of spinach.

Servings Provided: 4
Total Preparation & Cooking Time: 16-20 minutes
Total Macro Nutrients for Each Portion:
- Net Carbs: 3.5 g
- Fats: 14.6 g
- Total Protein: 18.3 g
- Calorie Count: 231

Essential Ingredients:
- Spicy Italian chicken sausages (4)
- Coconut oil (2 tbsp.)
- Onion (.5 cup)
- Purple cabbage (1.5 cups)
- Green cabbage (1.5 cups)
- Chopped fresh cilantro (2 tbsp.)
- Colby jack cheese (2 @ 1 oz./28 g slices)

Preparation Steps:
1. Start by removing the sausage casings and rough-chopping them. Shred the cabbage and chop the onions.
2. Dice the onion. Add the coconut oil, cabbage, and onion in a large skillet using the med-high setting for approximately eight minutes (the veggies should be tender). Blend the cheese and cover.
3. Extinguish the heat - let it rest five minutes as the cheese melts.
4. When it is time to serve—stir gently and add the cilantro.

Fiesta Lime Chicken

Servings Provided: 8 @ ½ breast each serving
Total Preparation & Cooking Time: 17 minutes
Total Macro Nutrients for Each Portion:
- Net Carbs: 5.6 g
- Fats: 6.2 g
- Total Protein: 31.4 g
- Calorie Count: 208.9

Essential Ingredients:
- Chicken breast (4 - cut in half)
- Garlic (3 cloves)
- Juice (1.5 limes)
- Salsa (1 cup)
- Reduced-fat ranch dressing (.25 cup)
- Cheddar cheese - reduced-fat (1 cup - shredded)

Preparation Steps:
1. Trim the chicken, making sure all fat and bones are removed.
2. Lightly spritz a skillet with cooking oil spray and heat using the medium-temperature setting.
3. Sauté the chicken for three minutes on each side. Mince and toss in the garlic.
4. Whisk the salsa, lime juice, and ranch dressing in a mixing container. Spread it over the top of the chicken. Simmer for an additional five minutes.
5. Garnish it with the cheese, cover, and cook until the chicken is no longer pink (4-5 min.).

Hasselback Marinara Chicken

Servings Provided: 6
Total Preparation & Cooking Time: 40 minutes
Total Macro Nutrients for Each Portion:
- Net Carbs: 2.6 g
- Fats: 18.3 g
- Total Protein: 18 g
- Calorie Count: 338

Essential Ingredients:
- Shredded mozzarella (.33 cup)
- Cream cheese (4 oz. or 110 g)
- Frozen spinach – thawed – liquid removed (10 oz. or 280 g pkg.)
- Chicken breasts (3)
- Olive oil (1 tbsp.)
- Tomato basil sauce (.66 or 2/3 cup)
- Mozzarella slices (3 oz. or 85 g)
- Salt & pepper (as desired)

Preparation Steps:
1. Set the oven to 400° Fahrenheit/204° Celsius.
2. Add the spinach and both types of cheese into a microwave-safe dish. Heat for two minutes and blend with the pepper and salt.
3. Slice the chicken tops horizontally without slicing 'all the way' through the breasts.
4. Stuff each piece with the filling mixture and brush with some oil.
5. Cook until the chicken reaches 165° Fahrenheit/74° Celsius (about 25 minutes).

Chapter 8

Lunchtime
& Dinner Seafood Specialties

Almond Pesto Salmon

Servings Provided: 2
Total Preparation & Cooking Time: 25 minutes
Total Macro Nutrients for Each Portion:
- Net Carbs: 6 g
- Fats: 47 g
- Total Protein: 38 g
- Calorie Count: 610

Essential Ingredients:
- Garlic (1 clove)
- Olive oil (1 tbsp.)
- Lemon (half of 1)
- Almonds (.25 cup)
- Parsley (.5 tsp.)
- Pink Himalayan salt (.5 tsp.)
- Atlantic salmon fillets (2 @ 170 g or 6 oz. each)
- Shallot (half of 1)
- Frisee lettuce (2 handfuls)
- Butter (2 tbsp.)

Preparation Steps:
1. *Make the Pesto*: Pulse the almonds, garlic, and olive oil in the food processor to form a paste. Add the parsley, salt, and juice of the lemon. Set to the side.

2. Dry the salmon fillets and flavor them with some pepper and salt.

3. Cook the salmon for four to six minutes (skin side down) in a lightly greased pan. Flip it and butter the pan to baste the fish for a minute or so. (The inside should be rare.)

4. Serve over some frisee with a dollop/scoop of pesto, slivered almonds, and shallots.

<u>*Bacon & Shrimp Risotto*</u>

Servings Provided: 2
Total Preparation & Cooking Time: 20-25 minutes
Total Macro Nutrients for Each Portion:
- Net Carbs: 5 g
- Fats: 9 g
- Total Protein: 24 g
- Calorie Count: 224

Essential Ingredients:
- Bacon (4 slices)
- Daikon winter radish (2 cups)
- Dry white wine (2 tbsp.)
- Chicken stock (.25 cup)
- Garlic (1 clove)
- Ground pepper (to your liking)
- Chopped parsley (2 tbsp.)
- Cooked shrimp (4 oz./110 g)

Preparation Steps:
1. Peel and slice the radish, mince the garlic, and chop the bacon. Remove as much water as possible from the daikon once it's shredded.
2. On the stovetop, warm a saucepan using the medium heat temperature setting. Toss in the bacon and fry until it's crispy. Leave the drippings in the pan and remove the bacon to drain.
3. Add the stock, wine, daikon, pepper, salt, and garlic into the skillet. Simmer until most of the liquid is absorbed (6-8 min.).
4. Fold in the bacon (saving a few bits for the topping) and shrimp along with the parsley. Serve.
5. *Tip*: If you cannot find the daikon, just substitute it using shredded cauliflower.

<u>*Broiled Oyster With Spicy Sauce*</u>

Servings Provided: 2
Total Preparation & Cooking Time: 20-25 minutes
Total Macro Nutrients for Each Portion:
- Net Carbs: 2 g
- Fats: 8 g
- Total Protein: 4 g
- Calorie Count: 102

Essential Ingredients:
- Oysters (1 dozen)
- Salt (.125 or 1/8 tsp.)
- Garlic chili paste - ex. Huy Fong's (1 tbsp.)
- Olive oil (1 tbsp.)
- Fresh basil (7-8 leaves)

Preparation Steps:
1. Warm the oven using the broil function.
2. Shuck the oysters.
3. Prepare the garlic chili paste, salt, and oil. Add the oysters and toss to coat them.
4. Sprinkle the leaves of basil onto an oven-safe baking dish and add the oysters
5. Empty the sauce into the dish.
6. Transfer the dish to the oven (top rack) and broil on high for two to three minutes, and serve right away.

Servings Provided: 8 cakes/2 per serving
Total Preparation & Cooking Time: 2 hours 25 minutes
Total Macro Nutrients for Each Portion:
- Net Carbs: 3 g
- Fats: 28 g
- Total Protein: 35 g
- Calorie Count: 28

Essential Ingredients:
- Butter (2 tbsp.)
- Celery (1 large rib)
- Mixed bell pepper (.5 cup)
- Shallot (1)
- Garlic (2 cloves)
- Sea salt and black pepper (as desired)
- Large egg (1)
- Worcestershire sauce (1 tbsp.)
- Hot sauce (1 tsp.)
- Low-cal mayo (2 tbsp.)
- Mustard - spicy brown (1 tsp.)
- Parmesan cheese (.5 cup)
- Crushed pork rinds (.5 cup)
- Lump crabmeat (1 lb./450 g)
- Olive oil (2 tbsp.)

Preparation Steps:
1. Warm a large skillet or sauté pan using the medium-temperature setting.
2. Chop/dice the celery, shallot, garlic, and peppers. Toss them into the skillet to sauté for about ten minutes.
3. Combine the mayo, egg, Worcestershire sauce, hot sauce, and mustard. Mix in the sautéd veggies and stir well.
4. Fold in the parmesan and pork rinds along with the crab

mixture.

5. Prepare a baking tray/large platter with a sheet of parchment paper and make eight patties.
6. Pop them in the fridge for one to two hours.
7. Warm a skillet (med-high temperature) and add the oil.
8. Fry the patties until browned - not flipping too frequently, or they may break apart.

<u>*Mahi-Mahi Fillets*</u>

Servings Provided: 4
Total Preparation & Cooking Time: 25 minutes
Total Macro Nutrients for Each Portion:
- Net Carbs: -0- g
- Fats: 13 g
- Total Protein: 21 g
- Calorie Count: 200

Essential Ingredients:
- Olive oil - divided (2 tbsp.)
- Butter - divided (3 tbsp.)
- Mahi-mahi fillets (4 @ 4 oz. or 110 g each)
- Kosher salt and black pepper (to your liking)
- Asparagus (1 lb. or 450 g)
- Garlic (3 cloves)
- Red pepper flakes (.25 tsp.)
- Lemon (1 sliced/zest and juice)
- Freshly chopped parsley (1 tbsp. + more for garnish)

Preparation Steps:
1. Prepare a large skillet using the medium temperature setting and add one tablespoon each of oil and butter.
2. Arrange the fish in the pan with a dusting of salt and pepper. Cook it until it is golden or about four to five minutes on each side. Plate it for now.
3. Pour the rest of the oil into the skillet. Toss in the asparagus with salt and pepper, and sauté until it's tender (2 to 4 min.). Transfer it to a plate.
4. Add the remaining two tablespoons of butter to the skillet. Mince and add the garlic, pepper flakes, lemon juice, zest, and parsley.
5. Take the pan off the burner and add back the fish, asparagus, and sauce to the skillet.
6. Serve with parsley as desired.

Wild Dill Salmon

Servings Provided: 4
Total Preparation & Cooking Time: 2 hours 10 minutes
Total Macro Nutrients for Each Portion:
- Net Carbs: 2 g
- Fats: 13 g
- Total Protein: 50 g
- Calorie Count: 341

Essential Ingredients:
- Water (2 cups)
- Wild-caught skin-on salmon (2 lb./910 g)
- Reduced-sodium vegetable broth (1 cup)
- Finely chopped onion (1)
- Thinly sliced lemon (1)
- Pepper and salt (as desired)
- Dill (3 sprigs)

Preparation Steps:
1. Combine all of the fixings in a slow cooker with the salmon on the bottom.
2. Prepare using the high setting for two hours. It's done once it flakes easily.

Chapter 9

Lunchtime & Dinner Pork
& Beef Specialties

Pork Favorites

Asian-Inspired Pork Chops
Servings Provided: 3
Total Preparation & Cooking Time: 20 minutes
Total Macro Nutrients for Each Portion:
- Net Carbs: g
- Fats: 5.5 g
- Total Protein: 12 g
- Calorie Count: 106

Essential Ingredients:
- Pork chops (3 thinly-sliced center cut)
- Bragg Liquid Aminos/Sub. for soy sauce/or another favorite keto-friendly (2 tbsp.)
- Black pepper (.5 tsp.)
- Garlic powder (.5 tsp.)
- Salt (1 pinch)
- Ginger (.5 tsp.)
- Minced garlic (2 tsp.)
- Diced onions (1 tbsp.)

Preparation Steps:
1. Mince the garlic and dice the onions. Toss everything into a zipper-type plastic bag. Shake the fixings.

2. Put the pork chops in a bag. Marinate for two to 24 hours in the fridge, turning the bag from time to time.
3. Discard the marinade and drain the meat.
4. Grill them for 12-15 minutes using the medium temperature setting or until the desired doneness.

Servings Provided: 12
Total Preparation & Cooking Time: varies - 3-4 hours
Total Macro Nutrients for Each Portion:
- Net Carbs: -0- g
- Fats: 20 g
- Total Protein: 23 g
- Calorie Count: 282

Essential Ingredients:
- Olive oil (1 tbsp.)
- Pork shoulder (4 lb./1.8 kg.)
- Broth or beef stock (.5 cup)
- Jamaican Jerk spice blend (.25 cup)
- Also Needed: Dutch oven/regular oven

Preparation Steps:
- Rub the roast well with oil and coat with the jerk spice blend.
- Use the dutch oven to sear the roast on all sides. Add the beef broth.
- Place a lid on the pot. Simmer for about four hours using the low heat setting. (You can also bake it for three hours at 375° Fahrenheit/191° Celsius.)
- Shred and serve.

Servings Provided: 6
Total Preparation & Cooking Time: 20 minutes
Total Macro Nutrients for Each Portion:
- Net Carbs: 3 g
- Fats: 18 g
- Total Protein: 15 g
- Calorie Count: 241

Essential Ingredients:
- Oil (1 tbsp.)
- Ground pork (1 lb./450 g)
- Chopped bell peppers (1 cup)
- Garlic (2 cloves)
- Chopped onion (.5 cup)
- Chopped baby spinach (4 cups)
- Shirataki noodles (2 pkg.)
- Grated parmesan cheese (.5 cup)

Preparation Steps:
- Prepare the Instant Pot using the sauté function and add the oil when hot.
- Toss in the pork and saute until slightly pink. Add the garlic, onions, peppers, and spinach. Scrape the browning bits from the bottom and secure the lid.
- Use the high-pressure setting for three minutes and quick-release the pressure. Empty the sauce over the noodles and garnish with the cheese.

<u>*Spicy Pork Brussels Bowls*</u>

Servings Provided: 4 or 1.5 cups
Total Preparation & Cooking Time: 30 minutes
Total Macro Nutrients for Each Portion:
- Net Carbs: 6 g
- Fats: 10 g
- Total Protein: 35 g
- Calorie Count: 280.5

Essential Ingredients:
- Olive oil spray
- 90% lean ground pork (1 lb. or 450 g)
- Red wine vinegar (2 tbsp.)
- Garlic (3 cloves)
- Smoky paprika (1 tsp.)
- Ancho chili powder (2 tsp.)
- Kosher salt (1 tsp.)
- Cayenne pepper (.25 tsp.)
- Freshly ground black pepper (.25 tsp.)
- Dried oregano (.25 tsp.)
- Ground cumin (.25 tsp.)
- Brussels sprouts (6 cups)
- Onions (.25 cup)
- Large eggs (4)

Preparation Steps:
1. Heat a large cast-iron or heavy nonstick skillet using the medium-temperature setting. Spritz with a bit of cooking oil spray.
2. Cook the meat, breaking it into small pieces.
3. Combine spices in a small mixing container.
4. Mince and add the garlic, season with spices and vinegar, and cook until browned and no longer pink in the middle (8-10 min.)

5. Set the fixings to the side on a plate.
6. Chop the onions and shred the brussel sprouts.
7. Add the brussels and onions to the skillet and cook using the high-temperature setting, occasionally stirring until the brussels start to brown and are tender (6-7 min.).
8. Return the pork to the skillet and toss everything (1-2 min.).
9. Warm a nonstick skillet and spray with oil. Once it's hot, cook the eggs - covered until the whites are just set, and the yolks are still runny (2-3 min.).
10. Serve them as desired.

<u>*Stuffed Pork Chops*</u>

Servings Provided: 4
Total Preparation & Cooking Time: 1 hour
Total Macro Nutrients for Each Portion:
- Net Carbs: 1 g
- Fats: 38 g
- Total Protein: 102 g
- Calorie Count: 778

Essential Ingredients:
- Bacon (3 slices)
- Thick-cut pork chops (4)
- Blue cheese (3 oz./85 g)
- Cream cheese (2 oz./56 g)
- Garlic powder (1 pinch)
- Black pepper & salt (to taste)
- Green onion (.33 cup)
- Feta cheese (3 oz./85 g)

Preparation Steps:
1. Set the oven temperature to 350° Fahrenheit/177° Celsius.
2. Lightly grease a baking tin.
3. Prepare the bacon, reserving the grease, and set it aside.
4. Mix the feta and blue cheese. Blend in the onions, bacon, and cream cheese. Mix well.
5. Split the pork's non-fat side and add the cheese mixture – closing with a toothpick or skewer. Sprinkle using salt, pepper, and garlic powder.
6. Sear them using the bacon grease in the skillet for 1.5 minutes per side.
7. Arrange the chops on the baking pan and cook for 55 minutes. Wait for the chops to rest for about three minutes.

Beef Favorites

Bacon Burger & Cabbage Stir-Fry

Servings Provided: 10
Total Preparation & Cooking Time: 20 minutes
Total Macro Nutrients for Each Portion:
- Net Carbs: 4.5 g
- Fats: 22 g
- Total Protein: 32 g
- Calorie Count: 357

Essential Ingredients:
- Ground beef (1 lb./450 g)
- Bacon (1 lb.)
- Small onion (1)
- Minced cloves of garlic (3)
- Cabbage (1 lb. - 1 small head)
- Black pepper (.25 tsp.)
- Sea salt (.5 tsp.)

Preparation Steps:
1. Dice the bacon and onion.
2. Combine the beef and bacon in a wok or large skillet. Prepare until done and store in a bowl to keep warm.
3. Mince the onion and garlic. Toss both into the hot grease.
4. Slice and toss in the cabbage and stir-fry until wilted.
5. Blend in the meat and combine. Sprinkle with pepper and salt to serve.

<u>BBQ Flank Steak</u>

Servings Provided: 8
Total Preparation & Cooking Time: 8 hours
Total Macro Nutrients for Each Portion:
- Net Carbs: 1 g
- Fats: 21 g
- Total Protein: 35 g
- Calorie Count: 342

Essential Ingredients:
- Flank steak (3 lb./1.4 kg.)
- Paprika (1 tsp.)
- Granulated garlic (1 tsp.)
- White pepper (1 tsp.)
- Salt (1 tsp.)
- Cayenne pepper (1 tsp.)
- Granulated onion (1 tsp.)
- Black pepper (1 tsp.)
- Coconut aminos (1 tbsp.)
- Water (.25 cup)
- Melted butter (2 tbsp.)
- Also Needed: Slow cooker

Preparation Steps:
1. Combine the seasonings, aminos, and melted butter. Rub into the steak.
2. Add the water to the cooker and the steak fixings.
3. Cook for eight hours (flip ½ through the cooking cycle).
4. Serve with some creamy spinach.

Servings Provided: 4
Total Preparation & Cooking Time: 15-20 minutes
Total Macro Nutrients for Each Portion:
- Net Carbs: 7 g
- Fats: 30 g
- Total Protein: 36 g
- Calorie Count: 455

Essential Ingredients:
- Small yellow onion (1)
- Ground beef (1.5 lb./680 g)
- Red enchilada sauce (.66 or 1/3 cup)
- Chopped green onions (8)
- Diced Roma tomatoes (2)
- Shredded cheddar cheese (4 oz./110 g)
- *Optional*: Freshly chopped cilantro (as desired)

Preparation Steps:
1. Use a wok or skillet to sauté the yellow onion and meat.
2. Drain the juices and add the green onions, tomato, and enchilada sauce.
3. Once it starts cooking, simmer for about five minutes.
4. Sprinkle your dinner using salt and cheese. Continue cooking until the cheese has melted. Stir in the cilantro.
5. Serve over chopped lettuce and a serving of sour cream - add the extra carbs and enjoy.

Ground Beef Eggplant Casserole

Servings Provided: 12
Total Preparation & Cooking Time: 4 hours 10-15 minutes
Total Macro Nutrients for Each Portion:
- Net Carbs: 5.7 g
- Fats: 12.8 g
- Total Protein: 15.9 g
- Calorie Count: 209

Essential Ingredients:
- Ground beef (2 lb./910 g)
- Cubed eggplant (2 cups)
- Olive oil (1 tbsp.)
- Salt (2 tsp.)
- Pepper (.5 tsp.)
- Mustard (2 tsp.)
- Worcestershire sauce (2 tsp.)
- Drained diced tomatoes (28 oz./790 g can)
- Tomato sauce (16 oz./450 g can)
- Grated mozzarella cheese (2 cups)
- Oregano (1 tsp.)
- Parsley (2 tbsp.)

Preparation Steps:
1. Sprinkle the salt over the sliced eggplant and let it rest for 30 minutes – or so. Add to a bowl and coat with the oil.
2. Combine the beef, pepper, salt, mustard, and Worcestershire sauce. Mash into the base of the pan and top it off with the eggplant. Spread out the tomatoes and sauce. Drizzle with the rest of the fixings.
3. Prepare on the high setting for two to three hours or low for three to four hours.

Chapter 10

Appetizer & Snack Specialties

Avocado & Bacon Caesar Deviled Eggs

Servings Provided: 1
Total Preparation & Cooking Time: 25 minutes
Total Macro Nutrients for Each Portion:
- Net Carbs: 2 g
- Fats: 30 g
- Total Protein: 16 g
- Calorie Count: 342

Essential Ingredients:
- Eggs (2)
- Mayonnaise (1 tbsp.)
- Dijon mustard (.25 tsp.)
- Squeezed lemon (.125 or 1/8 tsp.)
- Garlic powder (.25 tsp.)
- Himalayan pink salt (.125 tsp.)
- Smoked paprika (.125 tsp.)

Bacon-Avocado Filling
- Avocado (¼ of 1)
- Pastured bacon (1 slice

Preparation Steps:
The Filling:
1. Chop and avocado and bacon into ¼-inch pieces.
2. Toss the bacon into a skillet, and cook using the medium heat setting for three minutes or until browned.

3. Add the avocado and lower the temperature setting to low to simmer for an additional three minutes.

The Eggs:

1. Pour two quarts of water into a pot to boil. Adjust the temperature setting to low. Gently add the eggs to cook for eight minutes.

2. Plunge the eggs into an ice water bath for three minutes. Once chilled, remove the peels and slice them in halves - lengthwise.

3. Gently transfer the yolks, the lemon, mayo, lemon, salt, mustard, and garlic powder into a food processor. Pulse the mixture until it's creamy smooth.

4. Spoon the filling into the egg white and dust with the paprika.

<u>Bacon-Wrapped Brussel Sprouts</u>

Servings Provided: 12
Total Preparation & Cooking Time: 45 minutes
Total Macro Nutrients for Each Portion:
- Net Carbs: 1 g
- Fats: 4 g
- Total Protein: 4 g
- Calorie Count: 58

Essential Ingredients:
- Bacon (12 strips)
- Brussel sprouts (12 medium to large)
- Black pepper (as desired)

Preparation Steps:
1. Set the oven temperature at 375° Fahrenheit/191° Celsius.
2. Prepare a baking tray with a layer of foil.
3. Rinse and dry the sprouts using a paper towel.
4. Place the sprout on a slice of bacon and roll it until covered. Arrange them on the baking tray and season to your liking.
5. Bake them for 30 to 35 minutes. Serve using a toothpick as a handle.

<u>*Bacon-Wrapped Mushrooms*</u>

Servings Provided: 12
Total Preparation & Cooking Time: 20-25 minutes
Total Macro Nutrients for Each Portion:
- Net Carbs: 1.6 g
- Fats: 26.4 g
- Total Protein: 8 g
- Calorie Count: 275

Essential Ingredients:
- Strips of bacon (25)
- Portobello or white mushrooms (25)
- Black pepper & salt (as desired)

Preparation Steps:
1. Heat the oven to reach 400° Fahrenheit/204° Celsius.
2. Remove the stems from the mushrooms and wrap each cap with a bacon strip. Securely close with a toothpick.
3. Arrange each of the prepared treats on the prepared pan.
4. Bake for 15 minutes. Place on paper towels to drain. Serve or store for later.

<u>*Buffalo Chicken Jalapeno Poppers*</u>

Servings Provided: 5
Total Preparation & Cooking Time: Under 30 minutes
Total Macro Nutrients for Each Portion:
- Net Carbs: 4.6 g
- Fats: 19 g
- Total Protein: 16 g
- Calorie Count: 252

Essential Ingredients:
- Bacon (4 slices)
- Garlic - minced (2 tbsp.)
- Chicken - ground (8 oz./230 g)
- Buffalo wing sauce (.25 cup)
- Mozzarella cheese - shredded (.25 cup)
- Salt (.5 tsp.)
- Onion powder (.5 tsp.)
- Blue cheese - crumbled (.5 cup - divided)
- Unchilled cream cheese (4 oz./110 g)
- Jalapeno peppers (10 large)

To Serve:
- Ranch dressing
- Sliced green onions

Preparation Steps:
1. Heat the oven to 350° Fahrenheit/177° Celsius.
2. Cook, drain, and crumble the bacon. Mince the garlic. Prepare the jalapeno by cutting them into halves and remove its seeds.
3. Lay parchment paper or aluminum foil on a cookie sheet. Spread the half pieces of the jalapeno peppers on the foil or parchment paper.
4. Prepare a skillet using the medium temperature setting to cook the garlic, ground chicken, salt, and onion powder until the chicken is fully cooked (15 min.).

5. Dump this mixture into a big mixing container.
6. Combine the wing sauce with the mozzarella cheese and ¼ cup of the crumbled blue cheese. Put just a little bit of this mix into all of the pepper halves and top them with the crumbles of cooked bacon and the rest of the blue cheese.
7. Bake the jalapeno poppers for thirty minutes, and serve them with the ranch dressing and the green onions for flavor and garnish.

<u>*Cheese Quesadilla*</u>

Servings Provided: 1
Total Preparation & Cooking Time: 20 minutes
Total Macro Nutrients for Each Portion:
- Net Carbs: 10.3 g
- Fats: 14.2 g
- Total Protein: 23 g
- Calorie Count: 298.2

Essential Ingredients:
- Low-carb/low-fat wrap (1)
- Mexican blend cheese - ex. - Kraft shredded (.33 or 1/3 cup)
- Sour cream - full- fat (1 tbsp.)
- Salsa (2 tbsp.)
- Salted butter (about 1 tsp.)

Preparation Steps:
1. Lightly butter a wrapper and place it butter side down in a griddle or skillet.
2. Add cheese - leaving about a ¼-inch edge.
3. Wait and cook until the cheese is mostly melted.
4. Close the quesadilla by folding in half, cooking until browned and crispy.
5. Flip it over and cook the other side the same way. Slice it into three wedges and serve with sour cream and a low-sugar keto-friendly salsa.

<u>*Chicken Stuffed Avocado—Cajun Style*</u>

Servings Provided: 2
Total Preparation & Cooking Time: 5-10 minutes
Total Macro Nutrients for Each Portion:
- Net Carbs: 5.4 g
- Fats: 51 g
- Total Protein: 34.5 g
- Calorie Count: 638

Essential Ingredients:
- Cooked chicken (1.5 cups/7.4 oz.)
- Avocado (10.6 oz./2 med./1 large)
- Lemon juice - fresh (2 tbsp.)
- Mayonnaise (.25 cup)
- Cream cheese/sour cream (2 tbsp.)
- Onion powder (.5 tsp.)
- Salt & Cayenne pepper (.25 tsp. each)
- Garlic powder (.5 tsp.)
- Dried thyme & Paprika (1 tsp. each)

Preparation Steps:
1. Shred the chicken into small pieces.
2. Blend all of the ingredients—saving the salt and lemon juice until last.
3. Leave one-half to one-inch of the avocado flesh—scoop the middle. Remove the seeds.
4. Cut the center/scooped pieces of avocado into small pieces and fill each of the halves with chicken mixtures.

Chilled Prosciutto-Wrapped Asparagus Antipasto

Servings Provided: 16
Total Preparation & Cooking Time: 30 minutes
Total Macro Nutrients for Each Portion:
- Net Carbs: 0.7 g
- Fats: 3 g
- Total Protein: 2 g
- Calorie Count: 35

Essential Ingredients:
- Organic asparagus spears (16 large/450 g/about 1 lb.)
- Prosciutto (4 oz./110 g pkg.)
- Lemon juice (1 tbsp.)
- Fresh oregano - leaves only (1 tsp.)
- Fresh thyme - leaves only (1 tsp.)
- Flaky sea salt (.25 tsp. + more for finishing)
- Olive oil (2 tbsp.)

Preparation Steps:
1. Trim the ends from the spears and thinly slice the prosciutto.
2. Steam the asparagus spears for approximately eight to ten minutes or until crisp-tender and still bright green. Immediately immerse them into an ice bath for about 30 seconds until the cooking process stops, and the spears are cool to the touch. Drain and gently pat them dry.
3. Squeeze the lemon for juice. Meanwhile, whisk the oil, lemon juice, oregano, thyme, and sea salt. Set it aside.
4. Cut each slice of prosciutto in half across the middle (not lengthwise), so you have two equal sheets.
5. When the asparagus is ready, wrap one piece of prosciutto around each cooled asparagus spear and arrange it on a plate.
6. Drizzle the plate with the dressing and add a sprinkle of sea salt.
7. Store any leftovers covered in the fridge for several days. It's best if you can store the dressing separately.

Crispy Treats

Parmesan Chips

Servings Provided: 2
Total Preparation & Cooking Time: 15 minutes
Total Macro Nutrients for Each Portion:
- Net Carbs: 3.7 g
- Fats: 18 g
- Total Protein: 27.4 g
- Calorie Count: 277

Essential Ingredients:
- Turmeric (.25 tsp.)
- Basil (.33 tsp.)
- Thyme (.5 tsp.)
- Paprika (.5 tsp.)
- Parmesan cheese (6 oz./170 g)

Preparation Steps:
1. Grate the cheese into a mixing container and sprinkle with the spices. Stir well.
2. Program the oven to 370° Fahrenheit/188° Celsius.
3. Cover a cookie tray using a layer of parchment baking paper or foil.
4. Sprinkle the cheese mixture onto the tray to create the circles and add to the prepared tray.
5. Bake the chips for ten minutes and chill.
6. Serve hot or cold.

<u>Pizza Chips</u>

Servings Provided: 12 chips/4 chips per serving
Total Preparation & Cooking Time: 20 minutes
Total Macro Nutrients for Each Portion:
- Net Carbs: 0.6 g
- Fats: 7.8 g
- Total Protein: 7.4 g
- Calorie Count: 104

Essential Ingredients:
- Parmesan cheese (1 cup - grated)
- Pepperoni (12 slices)
- Dried oregano (1 tsp.)
- Optional for Serving: Low-carb pizza sauce

Preparation Steps:
1. Set the oven at 400° Fahrenheit/204° Celsius.
2. Line a baking tray with a silicone baking mat or sheet of parchment baking paper.
3. Spread the cheese in 12 circles across the baking sheet. They should be about one tablespoon, plus one teaspoon each. Bake them for two minutes.
4. Transfer the tray from the oven and sprinkle the oregano over the cheese.
5. Top each cheese circle with one slice of pepperoni. Bake until crispy (8 min.).
6. Remove the tray from the oven and use a paper towel to dab each chip to soak up the excess grease.
7. Place the chips onto a paper towel-lined cooling rack and cool them until they're crisp.
8. Serve with pizza sauce, if desired.

Spicy Roasted Nuts

Servings Provided: 6
Total Preparation & Cooking Time: 15 minutes
Total Macro Nutrients for Each Portion:
- Net Carbs: 2 g
- Fats: 29 g
- Total Protein: 4 g
- Calorie Count: 281

Essential Ingredients:
- Olive/coconut oil (1 tbsp.)
- Salt (1 tsp.)
- Walnuts/almonds/pecans (8 oz./230 g)
- Ground cumin (1 tsp.)
- Chili/paprika powder (1 tsp.)

Preparation Steps:
1. Combine each of the components in a skillet.
2. Prepare using the medium temperature setting until warm.
3. Cool as a delicious snack with your favorite beverage.
4. Store at room temperature in a closed container.

Chapter 11

Dessert Specialties

Almond Blackberry Chia Pudding

Servings Provided: 2
Total Preparation & Cooking Time: varies - up to overnight
Total Macro Nutrients for Each Portion:
- Net Carbs: 1 g
- Fats: 8 g
- Total Protein: 2 g
- Calorie Count: 109

Essential Ingredients:
- Chia seeds (.25 cup)
- Raw honey (drizzle)
- Sliced almonds (2-3 tbsp.)
- Vanilla almond milk (1.5 cups)
- Fresh blackberries (6 oz. or 170 g)

Preparation Steps:
1. Rinse and add the berries into a dish. Crush with a fork until creamy.
2. Pour in the raw honey, milk, and chia seeds. Stir well.
3. Refrigerate for several hours or overnight for the most delicious results.
4. Sprinkle with the almonds and several blackberries.
5. Serve any time.

<u>*Avocado & Chocolate Pudding*</u>

Servings Provided: 2
Total Preparation & Cooking Time: 30 minutes
Total Macro Nutrients for Each Portion:
- Net Carbs: 2 g
- Fats: 27 g
- Total Protein: 8 g
- Calorie Count: 281

Essential Ingredients:
- Cream cheese (2 oz./56 g)
- Ripe medium avocado (1)
- Natural sweetener – swerve (1 tsp.)
- Vanilla extract (.25 tsp.)
- Unsweetened cocoa powder (4 tbsp.)
- Pink salt (1 pinch)

Preparation Steps:
1. Combine the cream cheese with the avocado, sweetener, vanilla, cocoa powder, and salt into the blender or processor.
2. Pulse until creamy smooth.
3. Measure into fancy dessert dishes and chill for at least ½ hour.

<u>*Carrot Almond Cake*</u>

Servings Provided: 8
Total Preparation & Cooking Time: 60 minutes
Total Macro Nutrients for Each Portion:
- Net Carbs: 4 g
- Fats: 25 g
- Total Protein: 6 g
- Calorie Count: 268

Essential Ingredients:
- Eggs (3)
- Apple pie spice (1.5 tsp.)
- Almond flour (1 cup)
- Swerve (.66 or 2/3 cup)
- Baking powder (1 tsp.)
- Coconut oil (.25 cup)
- Shredded carrots (1 cup)
- Heavy whipping cream (.5 cup)
- Chopped walnuts (.5 cup)

Preparation Steps:
1. Grease the cake pan. Combine all of the fixings with the mixer until well mixed. Pour the mix into the pan and cover with a layer of foil.
2. Pour two cups of water into the Instant Pot bowl along with the steamer rack.
3. Arrange the pan on the trivet and set the pot using the cake button (40 min.).
4. Natural-release the pressure for ten minutes. Then, quick-release the rest of the built-up steam pressure.
5. Place on a rack to cool before frosting or serve it plain.

<u>*Coconut Bars*</u>

Servings Provided: 20
Total Preparation & Cooking Time: 10 min + chill time
Total Macro Nutrients for Each Portion:
- Net Carbs: 2 g
- Fats: 11 g
- Total Protein: 2 g
- Calorie Count: 108

Essential Ingredients:
- Shredded unsweetened coconut (3 cups)
- Liquid sweetener of choice (.25 cup)
- Coconut oil (1 cup)

Preparation Steps:
1. Line a pan with a layer of parchment paper.
2. Combine the ingredients to make a thick batter.
3. Pour into the pan and freeze until firm.
4. Cut into squares and store until you want a delicious snack.

<u>*Creamy Lime Pie*</u>

Servings Provided: 8
Total Preparation & Cooking Time: 25 minutes + chill time - 4 hours
Total Macro Nutrients for Each Portion:
- Net Carbs: 4.2 g
- Fats: 38.6 g
- Total Protein: 7 g
- Calorie Count: 386

Essential Ingredients:
- Almond flour (1.5 cups)
- Erythritol (divided - .5 cup)
- Salt (.5 tsp.)
- Egg yolks (4)
- Melted butter (.25 cup)
- Heavy cream (1 cup)
- Fresh key lime juice (.33 cup)
- Lime zest (1 tbsp.)
- Cubed cold butter (.25 cup)
- Vanilla extract (1 tsp.)
- Xanthan gum (.25 tsp.)
- Sour cream (1 cup)
- Cream cheese (.5 cup)

Preparation Steps:
1. Warm up the oven to 350° Fahrenheit/177° Celsius.
2. Add the butter to a pan to melt.
3. Mix the salt, half or .25 cup of the erythritol, and the almond flour. Slowly add the butter. Blend and press into a pie platter.
4. Bake for 15 minutes. Remove when it's lightly browned. Let it cool.
5. In another saucepan, combine the egg yolks, heavy cream, rest of the erythritol, lime zest, and juice.

6. Simmer using the medium-temperature setting until it starts to thicken (7-10 min.).

7. Take the pan from the hot burner and add the xanthan gum, vanilla extract, cold butter, sour cream, and cream cheese. Whisk until it's creamy smooth.

8. Scoop into the cooled pie shell. Use a layer of foil or plastic to cover the pie and place it in the fridge.

9. Note: You can serve after four hours, but it is better to wait overnight to enjoy the delicious treat.

Servings Provided: 15
Total Preparation & Cooking Time: 60 minutes
Total Macro Nutrients for Each Portion:
- Net Carbs: -0- g
- Fats: 8 g
- Total Protein: 2 g
- Calorie Count: 93

Essential Ingredients:
- Mashed avocado (8 oz./230 g)
- Baking powder (1 tsp.)
- Eggs (2)
- Cocoa powder (.5 cup)
- Keto-friendly sweetener of choice (.75 cup)
- Bacon (.25 cup)
- Dark chocolate chips - ex. ChocZero (.33 or 1/3 cup)
- Mayonnaise (1/3 cup)
- Vanilla extract (2 tsp.)
- Pan size Suggested: Baking pan (9x6 inches/23x15-cm)

Preparation Steps:
1. Set the oven temperature setting to reach 325° Fahrenheit/163° Celsius.
2. Prepare the pan with a layer of parchment baking paper and a misting of oil.
3. Fry the bacon until it's crispy and chop it to bits.
4. Toss each of the fixings - except for the chocolate chips and bacon in a blender. Puree the mixture until it's creamy smooth.
5. Fold in half of the bacon and half of the chocolate chips into the brownie batter. Empty it into the pan. Top it off using the rest of the bacon and chips.
6. Bake for 40-45 minutes. Then use a toothpick to test if the brownies are fully cooked. If it comes out clean, they're done; if

not, continue cooking for another five to ten minutes.

7. Once the brownies are thoroughly cooked, cool completely before cutting into 15 squares.

Lemon Mousse Cheesecake

Servings Provided: 1
Total Preparation & Cooking Time: 6-7 minutes
Total Macro Nutrients for Each Portion:
- Net Carbs: 1.7 g
- Fats: 30 g
- Total Protein: 4 g
- Calorie Count: 277

Essential Ingredients:
- Lemon juice (.25 cup/2 lemons)
- Cream cheese (8 oz./230 g)
- Salt (.125 or 1/8 tsp.)
- Lemon liquid stevia (1 tsp.)
- Heavy cream (1 cup)

Preparation Steps:
1. Use a mixer to blend the juice and cream cheese until it's smooth.
2. Mix in the remaining fixings till it's thoroughly incorporated.
3. Taste test. Add the mixture to a serving dish and sprinkle with some lemon zest.
4. Refrigerate until you are ready to serve it.

Low-Carb Cheesecake

Servings Provided: 5
Total Preparation & Cooking Time: varies - 2 hours 35 minutes
Total Macro Nutrients for Each Portion:
- Net Carbs: 2 g
- Fats: 17 g
- Total Protein: 4 g
- Calorie Count: 181

Essential Ingredients:
- Unchilled full-fat cream cheese (8 oz./230 g)
- Large eggs (2)
- Granulated stevia/erythritol blend (1.5 tsp.)
- Pure almond & vanilla extract (.25 tsp. of each)

Preparation Steps:
1. Set the oven temperature at 325° Fahrenheit/163° Celsius.
2. Prepare five of the muffin cups using cupcake liners.
3. Beat the cream cheese until it's smooth. Whisk in the eggs and remainder of the fixings.
4. Pour the batter into the cups and set the timer for 15 to 20 minutes, checking it at the 15-minute mark. They should be puffy and a little wobbly in the center when they are done.
5. Let them cool on the countertop before placing them in the fridge for two hours to chill before serving.

<u>*One-Minute Brownie*</u>

Servings Provided: 1
Total Preparation & Cooking Time: 5 minutes
Total Macro Nutrients for Each Portion:
- Net Carbs: 2 g
- Fats: 4 g
- Total Protein: 3 g
- Calorie Count: 129

Essential Ingredients:
- Chocolate chunks (1 tbsp.)
- Almond milk (.25 cup)
- Egg (1)
- Coconut flour (1 tbsp.)
- Cocoa powder (1 tbsp.)
- Stevia (1 tbsp.)
- Chocolate protein powder (1 scoop)
- Baking powder (.5 tsp.)

Preparation Steps:
1. Use lard to lightly grease an oven-safe ramekin or a microwave-safe bowl.
2. Whisk all of the dry fixings in a mixing container.
3. Mix in the chocolate chunks, egg, and milk, and mix it thoroughly till you have a smooth batter.
4. To Bake: Set the oven setting at 350° Fahrenheit/177° Celsius (15 min.) - OR - microwave it for one minute to enjoy.

<u>*Peanut Butter Fudge*</u>

Servings Provided: 20
Total Preparation & Cooking Time: 1 hour 10 minutes
Total Macro Nutrients for Each Portion:
- Net Carbs: 6 g
- Fats: 11 g
- Total Protein: 4 g
- Calorie Count: 135

Essential Ingredients:
- Coconut oil (3 tbsp.)
- Smooth peanut butter - organic - low-cal (12 oz./340 g)
- Coconut cream (4 tbsp.)
- Maple syrup (4 tbsp.)
- Salt (1 pinch)

Preparation Steps:
1. Prepare a baking sheet with a layer of parchment paper.
2. Melt the syrup and coconut oil using the medium heat setting on the stovetop.
3. Stir in the salt, coconut cream, and peanut butter. Dump the mixture into the prepared dish and chill in the fridge for at least one hour.
4. Slice into pieces and store or serve.

Pistachio Cookies

Servings Provided: 16
Total Preparation & Cooking Time: 45 minutes
Total Macro Nutrients for Each Portion:
- Net Carbs: 2 g
- Fats: 12 g
- Total Protein: 4 g
- Calorie Count: 135

Essential Ingredients:
- Melted butter (6 tbsp.)
- Chopped pistachios (.5 cup)
- Erythritol (.5 cup)
- Almond flour (2 cups)

Preparation Steps:
1. Toss each of the fixings into a mixing container.
2. Shape the dough into a long roll - cover with a sheet of plastic wrap.
3. Chill the log of dough for about ½ hour. Unwrap and slice into 16 portions.
4. Bake for 12 to 15 minutes. Cool slightly and serve as a delicious snack or dessert.

Servings Provided: 8
Total Prep & Cooking Time: 1 hr. + 45 min.
Total Macro Nutrients for Each Portion:
- Net Carbs: 5 g
- Fats: 26 g
- Total Protein: 8 g
- Calorie Count: 311

Essential Ingredients:
- Almond flour (1 cup)
- Libby's Canned Pumpkin (1 small can/15 oz./430 g)
- Baking powder (.5 tsp.)
- Coconut flour (.5 cup)
- Heavy cream (.5 cup)
- Stevia (.5 cup)
- Melted butter (1 stick/110 g)
- Large eggs (4)
- Vanilla (1.5 tsp.)
- Pumpkin spice (2 tsp.)

Preparation Steps:
1. Set the oven temperature setting to 350º Fahrenheit. Grease a pie plate with a spritz of coconut oil.
2. Combine all of the fixings in a mixing container until light and fluffy.
3. Dump the batter into the baking pan.
4. Set the timer and bake for approximately 70 to 90 minutes.

Strawberries With Coconut Whip

Servings Provided: 4
Total Preparation & Cooking Time: 20 minutes - varies
Total Macro Nutrients for Each Portion:
- Net Carbs: 10 g
- Fats: 31 g
- Total Protein: 4 g
- Calorie Count: 342

Essential Ingredients:
- Strawberries or other favorite berries (4 cups)
- Refrigerated coconut cream (2 cans @ 13.66 oz./390 g)
- 70% or darker unsweetened chopped dark chocolate (1 oz./28 g)

Preparation Steps:
1. Remove the solidified cream from the can of milk and set it aside for another time, saving the liquid. Pour it into a mixing container and whip it with a hand mixer until it forms stiff peaks (approximately five minutes).
2. Slice the berries and portion them into four dishes. Serve with a dollop of the cream. Garnish with the chopped chocolate and a few berries. Serve.

Strawberry Rhubarb Crumble

Servings Provided: 8
Total Preparation & Cooking Time: 50-55 minutes
Total Macro Nutrients for Each Portion:
- Net Carbs: 3.5 g
- Fats: 20.6 g
- Total Protein: 4.2 g
- Calorie Count: 230

Essential Ingredients:
Fixings Needed For The Filling:
- Strawberries (1 cup)
- Rhubarb (1 cup)
- Lemon juice (1 tbsp.)
- Steviva Blend or your favorite stevia/erythritol baking blend (1-2 tsp)
- Xanthan gum (.5 tsp.)
Fixings Needed For The Crumble:
- Walnuts (1 cup)
- Coconut flour (.5 cup)
- Flaxseed meal (.25 cup)
- Steviva Blend (or your favorite stevia/erythritol baking blend (.25 cup (+) 1 tsp.)
- Melted unsalted butter (6 tbsp.)
- Sea salt (.25 tsp.)
- Also Needed: 9-inch/23-cm glass pie plate

Preparation Steps:
1. Finely dice the rhubarb, walnuts, and strawberries.
2. Warm up the oven to 350° Fahrenheit/177° Celsius.
3. Grease the pie plate with butter and set it to the side for now.
4. Combine the filling ingredients and set them aside.
5. Combine .25 cup of the sweetener, coconut flour, walnuts, flaxseed meal, and sea salt in a mixing dish.

6. Add the butter and mix until it's crumbly. Set about .5 of a cup aside and add another teaspoon of sweetener.
7. Add the crumbled mixture to the pie plate and spread it out until flattened.
8. Pour in the fruit mixture over the crust. Sprinkle with the rest of the crust fixings.
9. Bake for 20 minutes with a layer of foil. Remove and cook the last 10 to 20 minutes until browned.
10. When done, place it in the fridge to set.
11. Slice and enjoy when it's firm.

Chapter 12

Your Special 21-Day Meal Plan
& Shopping Lists

"Once you believe in yourself, and you put your mind to something, you can do it."

Simone Biles

Your dieting plan is based on an average of 20 net carbs. You can easily substitute any of the items with another selection offered in your expansive recipes. I have also left room for extras during the day. It is recommended to consider speaking with a medical professional before making drastic changes to your current dieting methods.

Go slow at first and see how intermittent fasting affects your body. Plan on something light for breakfast while maintaining your goals throughout the day. The outlined meal plan focuses on basic meals; you can add sides and snacks according to your suggested net carb allotments daily.

And, remember, if you find this book useful in any way, a review on Amazon is always appreciated!

Your Special Plan - Week One

Day	Breakfast Time	Lunchtime	Dinnertime	Snack or Dessert
1	Green Smoothie 3 g	Chili Delight 5 g	Bacon & Shrimp Risotto 5 g	Coconut Bars 2 g
2	Almond Coconut Egg Wraps 3 g	Chicken & Bacon Chopped Salad 2 g	Chicken Sausage & Cabbage Melt 3.5 g	Pistachio Cookies 2 carbs each
3	Cinnamon Roll Smoothie 0.6 g	Broccoli "N" Cheese Soup 7 g	Broiled Oyster With Spicy Sauce 2 g	Leftover Coconut Bars 2 g
4	Avocado & Egg Fat Bombs 1.1 g	Crunchy Cauliflower & Pine Nut Salad 8 g	BBQ Chicken Casserole 4 g	One-Minute Brownie 2 g
5	Almond Lover Smoothie -0- g	Cauliflower & Kielbasa Soup 6 g	Almond Pesto Salmon 6 g	Low-Carb Cheesecake 2 g
6	Blueberry Muffins 5 g	Cheesy Salad Sandwich 4.5	Jamaican Jerk Pork Roast -0- g	Pumpkin Bread 5 g
7	Blueberry - Kefir Smoothies 6.6 g	Creamy Chicken Soup 2 g	Chicken Parmesan 3 g	Almond Blackberry Chia Pudding 1 g

Your Special Shopping List - Week One

Your shopping list includes all items for the first seven days. You will find it contains many items you probably already have in your pantry, fridge, or freezer. Look it over and group it according to your stock before heading to the market. You may also want to substitute ingredients for your meals; it's all your choice! You are ready!

*"By failing to prepare,
you are preparing to fail."*

Benjamin Franklin

Optional Ingredients:
- Collagen powder (2 tbsp.)
- Liquid stevia/your choice (3-5 drops)

Optional Garnishes:
- Bell peppers
- Lettuce Leaves
- Cucumber slices
- Oregano

Pantry:
- Unsweetened shredded coconut (3 cups)
- Chocolate chunks (1 tbsp.)
- Pork rinds (1 oz./28 g)
- Dry white wine (2 tbsp.)

- Cooked oats (.33 cup)
- Chia seeds (.25 cup)
- Almonds (5) + (.25 cup) + (2-3 tbsp.)

- Chopped pistachios (.5 cup)

- Raw honey (drizzle)
- Almond butter (2 tbsp.)
- Canola oil (.25 cup)
- Coconut oil (1 cup + 2 tbsp.)
- Olive oil (.5 cup + 3 tbsp.)
- MCT oil (2 tbsp.)

- Flax meal (1 tsp.)
- Almond flour (5 cups)
- Almond meal (2 tbsp.)
- Coconut flour (.75 cup + 2 tbsp.)

- Baking soda & powder
- Black pepper & salt +Sea salt
- Red pepper
- Garlic powder + Garlic seasoning (2 tbsp.)
- Jamaican Jerk spice blend (.25 cup)
- Konjac root fiber (2 tsp. or 8 g)

- Cumin (.75 tsp.)
- Bay leaves (3)
- Chili powder (2 tbsp.)
- Parsley (.5 tsp.)
- Hot smoked paprika (1 tsp.)

- Stevia (.5 cup)(1 tbsp.)
- Erythritol (.5 cup)
- Granulated sugar substitute - Swerve (1 tbsp.)
- Sweetener of choice (4 tsp.) + Liquid sweetener of choice (.25 cup)
- Granulated stevia/erythritol blend (1.5 tsp.)

- Pure almond & vanilla extract (.25 tsp. of each)
- Cocoa powder (1 tbsp.)

- Protein powder - Chocolate (1 scoop)

- Cinnamon (.75 tsp.)
- Allspice (.5 tsp.)
- Pumpkin spice (2 tsp.)

- Vanilla protein powder (2 tbsp.)
- Sugar-free vanilla extract (3.5 tsp.)
- White wine vinegar (3 tbsp.)
- Marinara sauce (.5 cup)

- Broth or beef stock (.5 cup)
- Chicken broth (2 cups) + (14.5 oz.)
- Chicken stock (.25 cup)
- Vegetable broth (1 cup)
- Tomato paste (170 g/6 oz.)

- Coconut cream (.5 cup)
- Worcestershire sauce (1 tsp.)
- Sliced black olives (2.25 oz./63 g)
- Keto bbq sauce (.75 cup)
- Keto ranch dressing (2/3 cup)
- Garlic chili paste - ex. Huy Fong's (1 tbsp.)
- Libby's Canned Pumpkin (1 small can)

Refrigerator:
- Organic eggs (19)
- Keto-friendly mayonnaise (.5 cup)

- Sour cream (2 tbsp.)
- Heavy cream (.75 cup)
- Almond milk (2.25 cups)
- Vanilla almond milk (1.5 cups)
- Coconut milk kefir (1.5 cups)

- Plain nonfat Greek yogurt (.33 cup)

- Butter (1 stick + 10 tbsp. + .5 oz.)
- Ghee (3 tbsp.)

- Colby jack cheese (2 @ 1-oz./28 g slices)
- Parmesan cheese (2 tbsp.)
- Shredded mozzarella (.5 cup)
- Sharp cheddar cheese (2 cups) + Cheddar cheese (1 cup)
- Cream cheese (8 oz. - full fat) + (regular - 12 oz.)
- Crumbled blue cheese (1 cup)
- Edam cheese (1 oz./28 g)
- Feta cheese (.25 cup)

Vegetables:
- Broccoli (1 cup)
- Cauliflower (1 head) + (.25 cup)
- Leeks/onion (2 tbsp.)
- Pine nuts (.25 cup)
- Rutabaga (1)
- Cucumber (1 cup)
- Iceberg lettuce (.5 cup)
- Frisee lettuce (2 handfuls)
- Romaine lettuce (9 cups) + Romaine/baby gem lettuce (2 oz./56 g)
- Tomatoes (3 medium) + Cherry tomato (1)
- Finely chopped chili peppers (.25 cup)

- Garlic cloves (4)
- Chopped onion (.75 cup) + Small onion (1)
- Chopped chives or spring onions (2 tbsp.)
- Shallot (half of 1)

- Purple cabbage (1.5 cups)
- Green cabbage (1.5 cups)
- Daikon winter radish (2 cups)

- Fresh basil (7-8 leaves)
- Fresh cilantro (2 tbsp.)
- Fresh parsley (4 tbsp.)
- Fresh ginger (1 tbsp.)

Fruit:
- Avocado (1.5)
- Medium banana (1)
- Fresh blackberries (6 oz./170 g)

- Fresh blueberries (.5 cup) + Fresh or frozen blueberries (.5 cup)
- Kiwi fruit (.5 cup)
- Freshly chopped pineapple (.33 or 1/3 cup)

- Lemon (half of 1)
- Lemon/lime juice (1 tbsp.)

Frozen:
- Frozen chopped spinach (230 g/8 oz.)

Meat & Seafood
- Cooked chicken breast/thighs (2 lb. or 910 g)
- Chicken breasts (1 lb.) + (1-2 cups - shredded)
- Frozen grilled chicken breast strips (22 oz./620 g)

- Bacon strips (10 pieces+ 8 oz./230 g)
- Ground beef 1.5 lb./680 g)
- Spicy Italian chicken sausages (4)
- Kielbasa sausage (1)
- Pork shoulder (4 lb./1.8 kg.)

- Oysters (1 dozen)
- Atlantic salmon fillets (2 @ 6 oz. or 170 g each)
- Cooked shrimp (4 oz. or 110 g)

Your Special Meal Plan - Week Two

Just remember, *"If you keep going, you won't regret it. If you give up, you will."*

Day	Breakfast Time	Lunchtime	Dinnertime	Snack or Dessert
1	Bacon & Avocado Omelet 5 g	Avocado Shrimp Salad 4 g	Bacon Burger & Cabbage Stir Fry 4.5 g	Leftover Pumpkin Bread 5 g
2	Pumpkin Spice Latte Smoothie -0- g	Buffalo Chicken Soup 4 g	Asian-Inspired Pork Chops 2.7 g	Strawberries With Coconut Whip 10 g
3	Baked Apples 5 g	Chicken Caesar Salad with Avocado & Bacon 3 g	Crab Cakes 3 g	Lemon Mousse Cheesecake 1.7 g
4	Spinach - Cucumber Smoothies 3 g	Chicken Yellow Curry 3 g	BBQ Flank Steak 1 g	Creamy Lime Pie 4.2 g
5	Breakfast Skillet 7 g	Greek Chopped Salad 2 g	Hasselback Marinara Chicken 3 g	Leftover Creamy Lime Pie 4.2 g
6	Strawberry Smoothie 5 g	Mexican Chicken Soup 5 g	Mahi-Mahi Fillets -0- g	Peanut Butter Fudge 6 g
7	Buttered Asparagus With Creamy Eggs 6 g	Grab & Go Jar Salad 4 g	Buffalo Wings 1 g	Leftover Peanut Butter Fudge 6 g

Your Special Shopping List - Week Two

*"Think of that feeling you'll get
when you've reached your goal weight."*

You may notice some of the items needed for week two are already stored in the fridge, pantry, or freezer.

Pantry:
- Crushed pork rinds (.5 cup)
- Almond flour (1.5 cups)
- Salt (.5 tsp.)
- White pepper (1 tsp.)
- Cayenne pepper (1.5 tsp.)
- Red pepper flakes (.25 tsp.)

- Cinnamon (2.25 tsp.)
- Instant coffee (1 tsp.)
- Cumin (1 tbsp.)

- Granulated garlic (1 tsp.)
- Garlic powder (1.5 tsp.)
- Granulated onion (1 tsp.)
- Ground coriander (2 tsp.)
- Ground ginger powder (2 tsp.)
- Paprika (1 tsp.)
- Dried thyme (1 tsp.)
- Pumpkin pie spice (.5 tsp.)
- Whey protein powder (1.5 scoops)

- Lemon liquid stevia (1 tsp.)
- Xanthan gum (.5 tsp.)
- Erythritol (divided - .5 cup)
- Keto-friendly sweetener (4 tsp.
- Coconut aminos (1 tbsp.)

- Pure maple syrup (1 tsp.)(4 tbsp.)
- Vanilla extract (1 tsp.)

- Chopped pecans (.25 cup)
- Almonds (8)
- Smooth peanut butter - low-cal (12 oz.)

- Coconut oil (6 tbsp.)
- MCT oil (4 tbsp.)
- Olive oil (4 tbsp.)

- Keto-friendly salsa of choice (1 cup)
- Marie's Creamy Caesar Dressing/your preference (6 tbsp.)
- Vinaigrette dressing (2 tbsp.)
- Hot sauce - ex. - Frank's Red (.25 cup/as desired)
- Keto-friendly mayonnaise (6 tbsp.)
- Spicy brown mustard (1 tsp.)

- Worcestershire sauce (1 tbsp.)
- Red hot sauce (.5 cup)(1 tsp.)
- Bragg Liquid Aminos/Sub. for soy sauce/or another favorite keto-friendly (2 tbsp.)
- Pumpkin (.33 cup - canned ok)

- Chicken stock (4 cups)
- Chicken broth (15 oz.)

- Mixed vegetables (preferably broccoli, and cauliflower (6 cups)
- Kalamata black olives (.25 cup)
- Tomato basil sauce (.66 or 2/3 cup)
- Crushed tomatoes (1 cup)
- Chunky salsa – ex. Tostitos (15.5 oz.)

- Coconut cream (4 tbsp.)
- 70% or darker unsweetened chopped dark chocolate (1 oz.)

Meat:
- Ground beef (1 lb./450 g)
- Flank steak (3 lb./1.4 kg.)
- Bacon (1 lb.) (1 slice) (1 cup crushed)

- Pork chops (3 thinly-sliced center cut)

- Grilled – pre-cooked chicken breast (1)
- Chicken drumettes/wingettes/wings (6)
- Organic ground turkey/grass-fed beef (.75 to 1 lb./340-450 g
- Chicken breasts (7) + (1.5 lb./680 g)
- Chicken thighs (1.5 lb.)

- Mahi-mahi fillets (4 @ 4 oz./110 g each)
- Shrimp (1 lb.) small-size

Refrigerator:
- Refrigerated coconut cream (2 cans)

- Seasoned tempeh (4 oz./110 g)
- Lump crabmeat (1 lb./450 g)

- Unsweetened almond milk (24 oz. or 230 g)
- Full fat coconut milk (1 can) + Coconut milk (1.75 cups)
- Heavy cream (2 cups)

- Butter - divided (9 tbsp.)(.5 cup)
- Ghee or coconut oil or butter (2 tbsp.)

- Large organic eggs (17)
- Plain Greek yogurt (.25 cup)

- Fresh parmesan cheese (1 cup) + (3 oz./85 g)
- Sour cream (2 cups)
- Shredded mozzarella (.33 cup) + Mozzarella slices (3 oz./85 g)

- Cream cheese (16 oz.) + (.5 cup)
- Crumbled blue cheese (.5 cup + more for serving)
- Pepper Jack/Monterey cheese (8 oz./230 g)
- Crumbled feta cheese (.25 cup)

Vegetables:
- Asparagus (24 oz./680 g) + (1 lb./450 g)
- Cabbage (1 lb. - 1 small head)
- Chopped romaine (2 cups)
- Spinach (2 handfuls)

- Celery (2 cups)
- Cucumber (2.75 oz./77 g)

- Garlic (8 cloves) + (2 tsp.)
- Ginger (2.5 tsp.)

- Cherry tomatoes (.25 oz./7 g)
- Leafy greens (.25 oz.)

- Celery (1 large rib)
- Red bell pepper (.25 oz.) + Mixed bell pepper (.5 cup)

- Shallot (1)
- Scallion (.5)
- Red onion (.25 cup)

- Onion: Medium (1) + Small (1) + Diced (1 tbsp.)

- Halved grape tomatoes (.5 cup)
- Tomato (1 small)

- Cilantro - fresh (2 tbsp.)
- Fresh parsley (1 tbsp. + more for garnish)

Fruit:
- Granny Smith apples (4 large)

- Ripe avocado (2) + (half of 1 small)
- Large strawberries (2)

- Lemons: juice (.25 cup/2 lemons) + (2 tbsp.)
  + (1 sliced/zest & juice)

- Freshly squeezed key lime juice (.33 cup) + (.25 cup)
- Lime zest (1 tbsp.)
- Strawberries or other favorite berries (4 cups)

Frozen:
- Frozen spinach (10 oz./280 g pkg.)
- Frozen vanilla yogurt (.33 or 1/3 cup)

Your Special Meal Plan - Week Three

"Think of that feeling you'll get when you've reached your goal weight."

Day	Breakfast Time	Lunchtime	Dinnertime	Snack or Dessert
1	Blueberry - Banana Bread Smoothie 4.7 g	Shrimp & Avocado Salad 4 g	Balsamic Chicken Thighs 4 g	Strawberry Rhubarb Crumble 3.5 g
2	Apple Cinnamon Muffins 3 g	Baked Zucchini Noodles With Feta 5 g	Wild Dill Salmon 2g	Leftover Strawberry Rhubarb Crumble 3.5 g
3	Chia Blueberry Coconut Smoothie 7.7 g	Steak Salad 1.5 g	Stuffed Pork Chops 1 g	Avocado & Chocolate Pudding 2 g
4	Leftover Apple Cinnamon Muffins 3 g	Cabbage Roll 'Unstuffed' Soup 3 g	Fiesta Lime Chicken 5.6 g	Carrot Almond Cake 4 g
5	Chocolate Smoothie 4.4 g	Vegetarian Club Salad 5 g	Ground Beef Eggplant Casserole 5.7 g	Leftover Carrot Almond Cake 4 g
6	Flaxseed Porridge 4 g	Leftover Cabbage Roll 'Unstuffed' Soup 3 g	Leftover Ground Beef Eggplant Casserole 5.7 g	Bacon Avocado Brownies -0- g
7	Mint Green Avocado Smoothie 5 g	Cauliflower Rice & Salmon Medley 5 g	Cheesy Bacon Chicken 1 g	Leftover Bacon Avocado Brownies -0- g

Your Special Shopping List - Week Three

You're almost there now; some of the items needed this week will probably already be in your stash!

Pantry:
- Coconut oil (.25 cup) + (2 tbsp.)
- Grapeseed oil (2 tsp.)
- Olive oil (6 tbsp.)
- Extra-virgin coconut oil (1 tbsp.)
- MCT oil (2 tbsp.)

- Chia seeds (5 tbsp.)
- Walnuts (1.5 cups)

- Almond flour (4 cups)
- Coconut flour (.5 cup)
- Golden flaxseed meal (3 tbsp.) + Flaxseed meal (.25 cup) +
- Flaxseed - plain or roasted is nutty-like (3 tbsp.)

- Dried basil (1 tsp.)
- Ground cumin (.25 tsp.)
- Parsley - dried (1 tsp.)
- Dried minced onion (2 tsp.)+ Onion powder (.5 tsp.)

- Apple pie spice (1.5 tsp.)
- Cinnamon (5 tbsp.)
- Nutmeg (1 tsp.)
- Cloves (.25 tsp.)
- Garlic powder (2 tsp.)
- Oregano (1 tsp.)
- Parsley (2.5 tsp.)

- Seasoning rub/seasoning salt or a mix of salt, garlic powder, onion powder, paprika (2 tbsp.)

- Banana extract (1.5 tsp.)
- Vanilla extract (2.75 tsp.Vanilla extract (.25 tsp.)

- Sweetener equivalent (2 tbsp.) sugar
- Optional: Protein powder/or another supplement
- Liquid stevia (10 drops)
- Xanthan gum (.25 tsp.)
- Natural sweetener – swerve (1 tsp. + .66 cup)

- Steviva Blend (or your favorite stevia/erythritol baking blend (.25 cup (+) 3 tsp.)
- Stevia extract (3-5 drops)
- Xanthan gum (.5 tsp.)
- Plain or chocolate whey protein (.25 cup)
- Cocoa powder (.5 cup) + Unsweetened cocoa powder (4 tbsp.)
- Unsweetened cacao powder (1 tbsp.)
- Dark chocolate chips - ex. ChocZero (1/3 cup)

- Sugar-free barbecue sauce - optional for serving
- Balsamic vinegar (.5 cup)
- Mustard (2 tsp.)
- Dijon mustard (1 tbsp.)
- Hot pepper sauce (.25 tsp./less if desired)
- Steakhouse seasoning (1 tbsp.)
- Wine vinegar (1 tsp.)
- Mayonnaise (1/3 cup) + (2 tbsp.)
- Reduced-fat ranch dressing (.25 cup)

- Japanese 7-Spice Shichimi - shichimi togarashi (2 tbsp.)
- Bragg's Aminos (.25 cup) + (4 tbsp.)
- Worcestershire sauce (5 tsp.)

- Beef broth (3 cups)
- Reduced-sodium vegetable broth (1 cup)

- Diced tomatoes (14 oz./400 g can) + (28 oz./790 g can)
- Tomato sauce (24 oz./580 g)

- Applesauce (4 tbsp.)

Refrigerator:
- Heavy whipping cream (.5 cup)
- Coconut cream (top of the full-fat coconut milk (.5 cup)
- Sour cream (2 tbsp.)
- Blue cheese (3 oz./85 g)
- Cheddar cheese - reduced-fat (1 cup - shredded)
- Cream cheese (4 oz.)
- Feta cheese (3 oz./85 g)
- Grated mozzarella cheese (2 cups)
- Swiss cheese - cubed (1 cup)

- Large eggs (13)

- Almond milk (.5 cup)
- Vanilla unsweetened coconut milk (2 cups)
    + Full-fat coconut milk (.75 cup)
- Unsweetened almond/cashew milk (1 cup)
- Coconut Milk - unsweetened (.5 cup)
    + Coconut milk or heavy whipping cream (.25 cup)

- Full-fat Greek yogurt/coconut
    or almond milk for vegan – dairy-free (1 cup)

- Almond or coconut butter (1-2 tbsp.)
- Butter (2.5 tsp.) + unsalted butter (6 tbsp.)
- Melted ghee (.5 cup)

- Feta cheese (8 cubes)
- Shredded cheddar (4 oz.)

- Salsa (1 cup)
- Pico de gallo (1 cup)
- Clamato juice (.5 cup - chilled)

Meat:
- Chicken breast (4 - cut in half) + (2.5 to 3 lbs. or 5 to 6)
- Chicken thighs (8/24 oz. approx.)
- Ribeye steak (1 @ 8 oz./230 g)
- Ground beef (2 lb.)+ 80/20 Ground beef (1.5 lb./680 g)
- Bacon (.25 cup) (3 slices) (.5 lb.)
- Thick-cut pork chops (4)
- Cooked shrimp (1.5 lb./680 g @ 31-40 per lb.)
- Wild-caught skin-on salmon (2 lb.)
    + Salmon fillets (4 @ 4 oz./110 g each)

Vegetables:
- Carrots (1 cup) + (1 small)
- Riced cauliflower (1 medium)
- Cucumber - diced (1 cup)
- Cubed eggplant (2 cups)

- Cherry tomatoes (.5 cup)
- Plum tomato (1)
- Chopped cabbage (1 medium)

- Romaine lettuce (3 cups) cut into pieces
- Green salad mix (2 cups)
- Orange bell pepper (1 medium)
- Zucchini (2)

- Garlic (9 cloves)

- Small onion (2)
- Green onion (.33 cup)

- Shallot (2 tbsp.)

- Cilantro (3 sprigs)
- Dill (3 sprigs)
- Large mint leaves (5-6)

Fruit:
- Ripe medium avocado (1) + (8 oz./230 g)

- Blueberries (.25 cup)
- Strawberries (1 cup)
- Rhubarb (1 cup)
- Lemon juice (1 tbsp.) + (1 tsp.)
- Thinly sliced lemon (1)

- Optional: Lime wedges
- Juice (1.5 limes) (2 tbsp.) (1 squeeze)

Frozen:
- Avocado (3-4 oz./85-110 g/half of 1) + (2 medium)

- Wild/frozen blueberries (2 tbsp.)
- Frozen blueberries (1 cup)

Chapter 13

Intermittent Fasting - The Final Words

Get Motivated Using Balance Exercises

> *"The only bad workout*
> *is the one that didn't happen."*

As you get older, you may not be as steady on your feet. Don't be discouraged; there are a few simple exercises you can perform in just a few minutes. It will bring back motivation once you realize you still have the opportunity to improve your gait.

All you need is the kitchen countertop or a steady chair for support. Let's give it a try!

• *Step 1: Try the Parallel Stance*: Relax and take a few deep breaths. Stand and extend your feet apart (about a hip's width). Do not hold onto the chair (it's there for backup), and keep the stance for ten seconds. If you did not wobble during that time, try step 2.

• *Step 2: Try the Semi-Tandem Stance*: Take a cleansing breath as you place one foot halfway in front of the other. Hold the pose for ten seconds - not holding a chair. It is similar to the stance used by an officer for a sobriety check. If you are a success, try the last pose.

- *Step 3: Try the Tandem Stance*: Take in a breath of fresh air. Place your mind in the tone that you are on a tightrope. Take the position (holding the chair for support if needed), standing with one foot directly in front of the other, and keep the pose for ten seconds. Slowly eliminate contact with a chair.

If you believe you are in good physical health, strength training is a crucial exercise. It can help support your muscle mass. Consider a bit of weight training with a set of light dumbbells. Try some of these basic exercises if your body can tolerate the positions.

FAQ Time

Check Your Medications

It's important to inform your doctor about your weight loss program. However, that doesn't mean you will need to eliminate the snacks. He/she may have prescribed some medicines that make you gain weight. These are a few to question:

- Insulin Injections: If taken in high doses, your insulin can impede weight loss. By consuming fewer carbs, you are substantially reducing the requirement of insulin. Again, ask your healthcare professional before you make any changes.
- Oral contraceptives
- Antidepressants
- Epilepsy drugs
- Blood pressure medications
- Allergy medicines
- Antibiotics

Supplements to Consider During IF

You will be embarking on a challenging diet method as you practice intermittent fasting. You may want to take a few supplements to prevent any possibility of deficiencies during the dieting phase.

- *Electrolytes*: You may experience headaches, fatigue, or nausea, sometimes called 'induction flu.' As you remove the carbs, your potassium and sodium (key electrolytes) are also removed. Taking a supplement will help with these issues.

- *Probiotics*: You can eat Greek yogurt, kefir, kimchee, or similar fermented foods. You can also take a supplement.

• *Greens/Veggie Supplements*: The best way to get the greens in your keto diet is through meals such as spinach in your eggs or a low-carb vegetable juice with a cheese snack. Have a salad with dinner. However, if you don't like greens, you can purchase a greens supplement. You can also add a measured scoop to a protein shake.

• *Potassium*: It is recommended to take supplements because potassium also leaves your body with salt. You can take 3 to 5 of the 99 mg tablets over-the-counter supplements.

• *Sodium*: You should receive at least one to two grams of extra sodium daily. Some of the pros accomplish this with bouillon cubes. Sea salt is a great option used in your diet plan.

• *Vanadium & Chromium*: These two are trace minerals essential to insulin production, which will stabilize your body's blood sugar level.

• *Malate or Magnesium Citrate*: Help your diet plan along with regularity (constipation) while activating over 76% of the enzymatic processes in your body. You can take between 400 to 600 mg each day.

It is suggested to contact your physician during each fasting phase to ensure your health remains on target. You may not need additional supplements if you have handled the meal planning phase in advance.

You need to remain diligent while on the kept-adapted diet plan since it can take several days to reach the keto state. One day of cheating can take your body a week to get back to ketosis. You may also gain water weight during the 'cheating' time.

If you are on the scales weekly and cheat, it is possible to see a four to six-pound weight gain even if you cheated five or six days ago. It will also take several more days for the weight loss to begin again.

Consistency begins with tracking the daily macros. The lists provide an additional layer of strictness to your diet. It makes you much more aware of the foods you consume in one day.

The book aims to teach how to promote longevity healthily, accelerate weight loss, reset metabolism, detox the body, and increase energy. I want the teachings in this book to easily be applied to the average person and *not just the elite athletic population.*

"Don't compare yourself to others. Compare yourself to the person from yesterday."

Conclusion

I hope you better understand how to proceed with your diet plan using your new copy of *Intermittent Fasting for Women Over 50*. Let's hope it was informative and provided you with all of the tools you need to achieve your goals - whatever they may be.

"Eat for the body you want,
Not for the body you have."

Here are a few last-minute tips about intermittent fasting and your approach.

1. Go Slow. Try two to three days of IF during the first week, and slowly increase the amount of time between meals.

2. Recognize the difference between wanting and needing to eat. Know how to recognize 'hungry' moments. Are you feeling a little shaky or weak? These are signs of - it is time to eat. You may need to eat more nutrient or calorie-dense food.

3. Stay Hydrated. Drink plenty of water and low-cal beverages, including tea or coffee. It's recommended to drink two to three liters of water or liquids daily.

4. Break your fast - steadily and slowly. Once it's time to eat, slowly chew your food so your digestive system can thoroughly process your food. It will allow you to know when you are full and help eliminate overeating.

5. Don't overeat. If you decide you don't want to do intermittent fast any longer, still use sensibility to keep yourself from sliding back into heavy feasting at every meal.

6. Enjoy balanced meals consisting of healthy fats, fiber, protein, and carbohydrates. You will see many selections in your meal plan and cookbook.

7. Test your plan. Choose which dieting technique works best for you and your schedule.

8. Adopt a workout schedule to keep your health moving forward and stay fine-tuned.

Finally, if you found this book useful in any way, a review on Amazon is always appreciated!